W9-BJE-509

ARTHRITIS

What You Need to Know

Johns Hopkins Editors
David B. Hellman, M.D.
Mary Betty Stevens Professor of Medicine
The Johns Hopkins University School of Medicine

Ada R. Davis, Ph.D., R.N.
Associate Professor of Nursing
The Johns Hopkins University School of Nursing

Editorial Director
Laura J. Wallace

Writer
Sara J. Henry

Johns Hopkins Office of Consumer Health Information
Ron Sauder, Director
Molly L. Mullen, Editor

Johns Hopkins USA assists out-of-town patients with any aspect of arranging a visit to the Johns Hopkins Medical Institutions—from scheduling appointments to providing guidance on hotels, transportation, and preferred routes of travel. The program has up-to-date information on clinical practices and is a resource center for maps, visitor guides, and other materials of interest to non-local patients. Client Services Coordinators in the Johns Hopkins USA offices are available Monday through Friday from 8:30 a.m. until 5:00 p.m. (Eastern). They can be reached toll-free at 1-800-507-9952 or locally at 410-614-USA1. You can also visit Johns Hopkins on the World Wide Web at http://hopkins.med.jhu.edu/.

Johns Hopkins
HEALTH

ARTHRITIS
What You Need to Know

TIME
LIFE
BOOKS

Alexandria, Virginia

The information in this book is for your general knowledge only. It is not intended as a substitute for the advice of a physician. You should seek prompt medical care for any specific health problems you may have.

TIME ®
LIFE
BOOKS

Time-Life Books is a division of Time Life Inc.

Time Life Inc.
President and CEO: George Artandi

Time-Life Custom Publishing
Vice President and Publisher: Terry Newell
Vice President of Sales and Marketing: Neil Levin
Director of Special Sales: Liz Ziehl
Editor for Special Markets: Anna Burgard

© 1999 The Johns Hopkins University
All rights reserved.
Published by Ottenheimer Publishers, Inc.
5 Park Center Court, Suite 300
Owings Mills, MD 21117-5001
JH008M L K J I H G F E D C B A

No part of this book may be reproduced in any form or by any electronic or mechanical means, including information storage and retrieval devices or systems, without prior written permission from the publisher, except that brief passages may be quoted for reviews.

First printing. Printed and bound in U.S.A. M L K J I H G F E D C B A

Time-Life is a trademark of Time Warner Inc. U.S.A.

ISBN: 0-7370-1600-0

Library of Congress Cataloging-in-Publication Data
Henry, Sara J.
    Arthritis : what you need to know / by Sara J. Henry.
        p.   cm. — (Johns Hopkins health)
    ISBN 0-7370-1600-0 (pbk. : alk. paper)
    1. Arthritis Popular works.   I. Title.   II. Series.
RC933.H46   1999
616.7'22—dc21   99-26956
                                                                      CIP

Books produced by Time-Life Custom Publishing are available at special bulk discounts for promotional and premium use. Custom adaptations can also be created to meet your specific marketing goals. Call 1-800-323-5255.

CONTENTS

INTRODUCTION. 1

1. WHAT IS ARTHRITIS?. 5
    When Things Go Wrong 6
    What Types of Arthritis Are There? 7
    Who Gets Arthritis? 9
    The Big Two: OA and RA. 10
    What Causes Arthritis? 12
    What Does Treatment Involve? 16
    Can I Prevent Arthritis? 17
    Coping with a Chronic Condition 19
    Struggling with Arthritis 20
    Working with Your Doctors. 21

2. HOW TO TELL IF YOU HAVE ARTHRITIS 23
    When Do You Need to See a Doctor? 24
    How Will Arthritis Make You Feel? 24
    How Your Doctor Diagnoses Arthritis. 26
    A Look at Other Types of Arthritis 30
    How to Prepare for Your Doctor Visit 34

3. FINDING MEDICAL CARE. 37
    Why You Shouldn't Wait It Out 37
    Whom Do You Need to See?. 38
    Specialists You May Encounter 39
    Other Health Care Professionals Who Can Help You 40
    Effective Communication with
        Your Health Care Professional. 42
    How *Not* to Get the Most Out of Your Doctor 45

4. FIGHTING ARTHRITIS WITHOUT DRUGS............... 47
   Educate Yourself—and Others...................... 48
   Hot and Cold Treatments 48
   Exercise: Feeling Better in a Fitter Body 50
   The Value of Rest 57
   What Physical Therapy Can Mean to You............. 58
   What About "Unconventional" Treatments?............ 60

5. WHAT YOU EAT CAN MAKE A DIFFERENCE 67
   Is There a Food Culprit? 67
   How to Avoid Osteoporosis........................ 69
   Fatty Acids and You............................. 73
   The Arthritis Diet............................. 73
   Ten Tips to Make Eating Well Easy 76
   Interactions with Your Medications 78

6. MEDICATIONS TO FIGHT ARTHRITIS 81
   Over-the-Counter Medication May Be the Answer....... 82
   Tingly Salves and Such 83
   The Next Step for OA............................ 84
   Treating Inflammatory Diseases.................... 88
   Aspirin Can Be Your Friend 89
   Reducing the Side Effects of NSAIDs................. 90
   The Scoop on the SAARDs 93

7. WHAT IF YOU HAVE OTHER TYPES OF ARTHRITIS?........ 101
   Bursitis and Tendinitis.......................... 101
   Fibromyalgia 104
   Gout and Pseudogout 107
   Juvenile Rheumatoid Arthritis 111
   Lupus 112
   Lyme Disease 115
   Polymyalgia Rheumatica and Giant Cell Arteritis 117
   Sjögren's Syndrome 120
   Inflammatory Arthritis and the Spine 121

8. WHEN SURGERY IS NECESSARY 125
   What Is Arthroscopy? 126
   What Is a Synovectomy? 127
   A Look at Joint Replacement. 128
   A Closer Look at Hips and Knees 129
   Which Type of Joint?. 132
   A Look at Other Procedures 133
   The Nitty Gritty of Surgery. 135
   Things to Do Before You Leave Home 137
   How to Avoid Pocketbook Shock 139
   What to Expect After Surgery. 140

9. HELPING YOURSELF LIVE WITH ARTHRITIS 143
   Give Your Joints a Helping Hand 143
   Using Splints and Other Supports 144
   You're Not Alone. 147
   Finding the Right Shoes and Orthotics 148
   Arthritis and Your Love Life 149
   Rethink Your Routines. 149
   Day-to-Day Living Made Easier 152
   Make Some Changes at Work 154
   What If You Get Pregnant? 156
   Changing Your Outlook. 158

10. AN EXERCISE PROGRAM FOR YOU. 161
    Planning Your Attack 162
    All About Walking 164
    All About Stretching. 165
    All About Swimming. 169
    All About Water Workouts 170
    All About Bicycling. 172
    All About Weight Lifting 174

11. THE FUTURE OF ARTHRITIS TREATMENT 177
   Repairing and Replacing Cartilage 178
   Other Areas Under Study 179
   Unlocking the Inflammation Puzzle 180
   How to Keep Up with the Latest News 181

INTRODUCTION

Arthritis can be the gnarled fingers of your grandmother, no longer able to do the knitting she loves. The pain in your spouse's knees that keeps you from taking your companionable neighborhood stroll together after dinner. Or the early morning stiffness that prevents you from bouncing cheerfully out of bed and into the day.

These are the types of problems experienced by nearly 40 million Americans, all of whom suffer from one form of arthritis or another. Untreated, this disease can diminish your ability to do simple tasks, make you lose days from work, or quit work altogether. It can affect day-to-day life, relationships, jobs, hobbies, travel, and the overall quality and length of your life.

Yet the word "arthritis" covers many conditions. The most common, osteoarthritis, damages the cartilage that cushions your joints and can leave you unable to walk without pain. The second most common form, rheumatoid arthritis, leaves your joints painful and swollen and, when untreated, can be crippling. Other types of arthritis and related conditions—polymyalgia rheumatica, fibromyalgia, bursitis and tendinitis, gout, and the arthritis of Lyme disease, for example—can be painful, exhausting, frustrating, and depressing. Still other types can damage your heart, lungs, kidneys, or eyes.

Arthritis can rob you of your mobility, your independence, and sometimes your very pleasure in life.

But it doesn't have to be that way.

You can fight back. You can take charge of your life and your arthritis and hold back its ability to control you.

The first tool you need is knowledge. You need to know exactly which type of arthritis you have and what treatment options are available. There is seldom just one treatment: As much as we all wish it were otherwise, there is no magic pill that makes arthritis disappear. Medications can help, but you can fight arthritis in many ways. You may make changes in how you walk and move and how you do minor tasks around the home or at work. You may start making time for an exercise program or improve your diet. And you'll want to learn the latest techniques of pain management and ingenious ways to lessen strain on damaged joints.

So in this book we break things down: We explain the different types of arthritis, explore how you can treat the disease without drugs, discuss alternative treatments, and tell you what works and what doesn't—and which treatments doctors aren't sure about yet. We tell you how to get what you want and need from your doctor, review medical tests, and examine the pros and cons of various medications. And because arthritis can drag you into depression, we guide you to help for that, too.

You can't fight arthritis alone, however: You need sound health care. But unfortunately, medical treatment of arthritis is an inexact science. Medical tests can be confusing, and the drugs available and their side effects mind-boggling. This book tells you not only how to find the best health care professionals—from family doctors to rheumatologists to nutritionists to physical therapists—but also how to work effectively with them and benefit most from the process.

We explain medical tests and talk about medication. We discuss the most common drugs and tell you how they work, what their drawbacks are, and what you can expect when you take them. We detail the surgical options available and give you practical help—such as how you may need to rearrange things at home before surgery, what to pack for the hospital, and how to speed your recovery once you're back home.

Two important ways to prevent and treat some forms of arthritis are diet and exercise. We show you a style of eating that will ease your battle, then give you tips on building gentle arthritis-fighting exercises and stretches into your daily life. We tell you the experts' tricks for living with arthritis—how to open doors, get out of bed, and sit down without pain—and explore some of the clever gadgets available that can make your day-to-day life infinitely easier.

This is an exciting time in arthritis treatment. Research is exploding, and innovative treatments and ways of dealing with arthritis are popping up. But sometimes the reports can be confusing. You may hear one thing from your neighbor, read another in a magazine article, and then hear something on the news that seems to contradict them both. You need a reliable source you can trust, one that takes into account the very real needs and concerns of the person who must deal with arthritis every day.

The Johns Hopkins University (including its world-renowned schools of medicine, nursing, and public health) and the closely related Johns Hopkins Health System are well known for their commitment to medical research, education, and patient care. For the past eight years, The Johns Hopkins Hospital has been ranked the number one hospital in the United States in an annual survey conducted by *U.S. News and World Report*.

In this book Johns Hopkins presents a comprehensive, clearly written guide to the challenge of life with arthritis. When it comes to health advice, you want both expert knowledge and compassionate guidance, and that's precisely what you'll find here. The information in this book is based on the latest research and years of experience of the finest health professionals anywhere. You can be assured that what you read within these pages is information you can trust and just what you need at your side in your fight against arthritis.

CHAPTER 1

What Is Arthritis?

Your hip aches every time you settle into your favorite armchair. Your spouse's knee is beginning to twinge on every trip up and down the stairs. Your uncle's fingers are so swollen and painful he has given up whittling. And your mother's neck and shoulders ache so painfully she couldn't dance at your son's graduation.

All these conditions are arthritis.

But they're different types of arthritis. And not only does each type need a specific treatment, but also, because no two people are alike, what works well for you may not work well for your neighbor or friend with the same ailment.

One person may need a change of diet or a change in work habits. Another may simply need to rest more often and take aspirin occasionally. A third may need antibiotics right away or strong drugs to prevent becoming disabled later in life. Still others may need completely different types of treatment.

That's why you need to know the type of arthritis you have, know your treatment options, and know yourself. With the help of your doctor and other health care practitioners, you can find a treatment plan that fits you, your life, and your condition.

You should be in charge of your health—not the other way around.

When Things Go Wrong

When you think about it, our bodies are amazingly mobile. They're constructed so that we can easily bend our knees, ankles, elbows, wrists, and fingers. Some joints move in many directions, such as our hips, which have a ball-and-socket arrangement that allows fluid movement. Others are elegant hinges.

One thing that helps our joints move smoothly is a spongy material at the ends of the bones called cartilage, which cushions the bones and keeps them from rubbing against each other. You may have seen cartilage in a piece of chicken—that tough, springy, translucent material—and our cartilage is somewhat similar. Another thing that helps is the synovial membrane, a lining in the joint. This membrane pumps out a lubricating fluid that works somewhat like the oil you put in your car. Without this fluid and cartilage, we'd be like the Tin Woodman when he rusts up. In fact, if problems develop with your cartilage or joint lining, you may begin to *feel* like the Tin Woodman after a thunderstorm—with the oil can just out of reach.

Problems occur when parts of our joints begin to wear out from overuse or simple wear and tear, such as when the cartilage becomes chipped or torn. Or the synovium can become swollen and then damage the nearby cartilage, ligaments, and bones. Still other pains may be caused by problems such as tears or strains in the muscles, tendons, and ligaments that support the joint.

We call many of these problems arthritis: "arth" means joint, and "itis" means swollen or inflamed, so the word just means inflammation of a joint or joints. The inflammation will often make the joint swollen or red, but in some cases no swelling is present.

It's important to understand that pain around a joint is not always arthritis, however. Other causes of inflammation around a joint may produce pain that feels just like arthritis but is not. Some other causes of this pain can be conditions like bursitis, tendinitis, polymyalgia rheumatica (all of which we'll discuss in detail). Your doctor will detect the true culprit by taking your medical history and giving you a physical examination.

WHAT TYPES OF ARTHRITIS ARE THERE?

There are over 100 forms of arthritis. Doctors tell them apart by determining which joints or structures of the body are affected. In some types of arthritis, other parts of the

---

POSSIBLE SOURCES OF JOINT PAIN

Feeling pain in your joints? Don't be too quick to diagnose yourself. Several areas of the joint can develop problems and cause pain. Damage to cartilage on the ends of the bones of the joint—either from wear-and-tear or from trauma— causes osteoarthritis. An inflamed synovium, the membrane between bones that meet in the joint, may mean rheumatoid arthritis. An inflammation of the bursa, the small, fluid-filled sac that cushions a joint, can be bursitis. Or the tendons, the string-like structures that connect muscles to bones, can become inflamed, which is called tendinitis. The only way to know for sure what's causing your pain is to see your doctor.

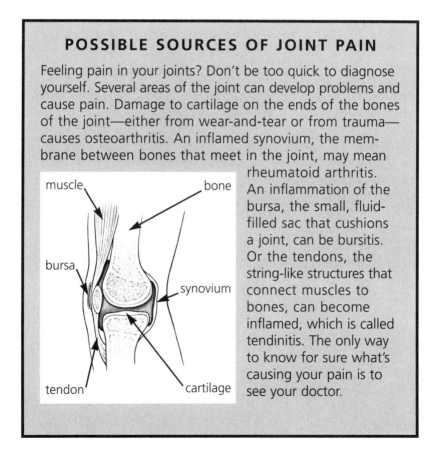

---

body also come into play. Osteoarthritis, for example, damages only the joints. Rheumatoid arthritis, however, affects not only the joints but also other systems of the body (particularly the immune system). And at the extreme end of the arthritis spectrum, the disease called lupus affects multiple organs, with the joints happening to be one.

Of all the types of arthritis and related ailments, two affect us the most: osteoarthritis and rheumatoid arthritis. (You may find these abbreviated as OA and RA in some books or articles.) Many people confuse the two, possibly because our grandparents used to refer to their aches and pains as rheumatism, while often they actually had osteoarthritis. While osteoarthritis is far more common, rheumatoid arthritis is more difficult to treat and can have a far greater impact on your life, so it's crucial to know the difference.

Some other types of arthritis affect the joint in similar ways. Many other arthritic conditions, however, affect the joint indirectly by damaging nearby body parts, such as the muscles, tendons, and ligaments that support the joint, or by causing swelling of the bursae, fluid-filled sacs that cushion the joint. While some of these conditions aren't technically arthritis because they don't involve swelling of the joint itself, they're often lumped together with it because they all affect the joint in one way or another.

The most common types of arthritis and related conditions, which are covered in this book, include lupus, gout, Lyme arthritis, bursitis, fibromyalgia, polymyalgia rheumatica, and giant cell arteritis. We'll also discuss psoriatic arthritis, Sjögren's syndrome, arthritis of inflammatory bowel disease, ankylosing spondylitis, and Reiter's syndrome.

WHO GETS ARTHRITIS?

Unfortunately, most of us get arthritis. More Americans have arthritis than any disease other than high blood pressure. The Arthritis Foundation estimates that nearly 40 million suffer from arthritis of some kind, and as the population ages in the next two decades, that number is likely to skyrocket. With advances in medicine and improved diet and work conditions, we live a lot longer than we did in pioneer days. The downside of this longevity is that our bodies aren't designed to function flawlessly for all these years. And sometimes we aren't as careful with our bodies as we could be.

Although we may not be aware of it yet, by the time we hit 40, nearly 9 out of 10 of us will have some osteoarthritis in the joints that carry body weight, most likely our knees and hips. Today, 15 million to 25 million Americans have osteoarthritis.

About seven million Americans have rheumatoid arthritis. That's roughly equivalent to every man, woman, and child who lives in the state of North Carolina. While rheumatoid arthritis can hit anytime—there's even a juvenile form that small children get—it most often strikes between the ages of 20 and 50. Women tend to have rheumatoid arthritis more often than men, which suggests a hormonal or genetic connection.

Other forms of arthritis, such as gout, Lyme arthritis, fibromyalgia, and polymyalgia rheumatica, occur far less frequently, although some of these have been on the rise. For instance, Lyme disease, once limited largely to a few northeastern states, has now been found in almost every state. Some others, such as polymyalgia rheumatica, have increased in number as these diseases become better known and methods of detecting them have improved.

THE BIG TWO: OA AND RA

Both osteoarthritis (OA) and rheumatoid arthritis (RA) involve pain and swelling in the joints, but there the similarity ends. The inflammation or swelling of rheumatoid arthritis is much more severe than the swelling that can occur in osteoarthritis. With osteoarthritis, the basic problem is the breakdown of cartilage and sometimes bone. It can be so uncomfortable that the pain keeps you from moving your joint. The nearby muscles become weak because you aren't exercising them enough, and the joint can "freeze up." While osteoarthritis, unlike rheumatoid arthritis, won't shorten your life, without proper care it may drastically limit your activity and change your lifestyle—which of course can be pretty depressing. Fortunately, treatment can make an enormous difference.

Rheumatoid arthritis is a much more serious disease that must be treated promptly to avoid permanent damage. Untreated, it can damage your joints and lead to serious complications, even in other parts of your body. With this disease, your immune system, which normally protects your body and helps you recover from illnesses goes awry, attacking your joints and causing the membrane that lines them to swell and thicken. Cartilage and bone may be destroyed, and in severe cases, the inflammation can affect the covering of the heart, small blood vessels, lungs, eyes, mouth, lymph glands, or spleen. As if this isn't bad enough, the disease also can make you feel rotten. You may lose your appetite, hurt all over, run a fever, and feel tired all the time.

What exactly happens in rheumatoid arthritis? For reasons no one understands completely, your immune system causes your body to attack itself. Think about allergies: For some reason your body sees the allergen—mold or pollen or peanuts or whatever—as a threat to the body. It kicks into full-scale battle mode, fighting an enemy that doesn't exist.

Something similar happens in rheumatoid arthritis. Some researchers believe a virus or bacterium gets into your joint and triggers the process. Whatever the cause, your immune system, normally a well-tuned and helpful setup, kicks into attack mode. Special white blood cells band together to fight the infections or invaders such as bacteria. These cells produce healing and infection-fighting substances, which also happen to cause inflammation during

IS IT OSTEOARTHRITIS OR RHEUMATOID ARTHRITIS?

While only test results and a doctor's diagnosis can verify what you're dealing with, there are general signs.

Osteoarthritis:
- usually begins after age 40
- develops slowly, over a period of years
- may affect only joints on one side of the body
- usually affects main weight-bearing joints, such as the knees and hips (rather than elbows, shoulders, or ankles)
- may affect the last joints of your fingers, the ones closest to your fingernails
- usually leaves joints "cool"—you won't see redness or swelling
- usually won't affect your overall health

Rheumatoid arthritis:
- may begin by age 25 and usually before age 50
- may develop suddenly, during a period of weeks or months
- usually affects joints on both sides of the body
- usually causes inflammation—joints are red, warm, and swollen
- usually affects small joints of the hand, foot, and wrist or elbow, shoulder, or ankle
- may cause overall tiredness, weight loss, and fever

the battle. When the battle is won and the wound is healed or the infection cured, normally your white blood cells calm down and the inflammation gradually goes away.

Unfortunately, in rheumatoid arthritis and other inflammatory diseases, there's no "off" switch to tell your body the war is over. The protective cells are in battle mode with nothing to sound the all clear, so you end up with inflamed, swollen, painful joints.

In some people, not much happens besides the swelling that makes joints uncomfortable. In others, however, the disease gets worse. The membrane that lines the joint—the synovium—gets thick and rough. White blood cells gather and release enzymes that inflame the membrane and cause it to accumulate fluid. Sometimes the synovium starts to grow, even over the cartilage of the joint, and this growth in turn produces enzymes that erode the cartilage and bone.

For some people, without careful treatment rheumatoid arthritis can be crippling. Hands, feet, and arms may become not only stiff and painful, but also deformed. And rheumatoid arthritis can damage the lungs, heart, or eyes as well. Again, however, good medical treatment can forestall the worst damage in most cases.

What Causes Arthritis?

There are many different causes of arthritis. Some are genetic, some lifestyle-related, and some environmental, such as bacteria and viruses. (The arthritis of Lyme disease, for instance, is caused by bacteria from an infected tick.) Still other causes aren't yet known or completely understood.

For osteoarthritis, the major cause is often described as wear and tear. But the true cause is not quite so simple as that expression might make it seem. The cartilage in your joints is living tissue, and its cells are continually undergoing changes and repair. For reasons we don't yet fully understand, as we get older our cartilage is more likely to become damaged and gradually lose its ability to heal itself. And the bone in our joints breaks down and re-forms itself, too, by forming small projections called spurs that function almost like nature's own splints. (We'll discuss splints in more detail in chapter 9.)

If you're overweight, your knee and hip joints are toting more than they were built to carry, and they wear out a little faster. And if you do an activity that requires your knees or hips to do a certain motion over and over, such as playing football or climbing stairs many times a day, those joints undergo extra stress as well. Inherited or genetic factors can also play a role in the development of osteoarthritis.

There are two basic types of osteoarthritis, primary and secondary.

Primary osteoarthritis. The damage occurs over decades and is caused by stress on the joint: Some is just from everyday living, but being overweight puts extra stress on your knees and hips and makes them more likely to become arthritic. What happens in this disease? As we've said, when cartilage is young and healthy, it rebuilds itself, just as you grow new skin cells to replace the old. Eventually, however, you break down more cartilage than you can build. Your protective cartilage's smooth surface gradually becomes roughened, then pitted with tiny holes. The bone underneath is no longer adequately cushioned, and small bone spurs or "lips" form at the edge of the joint in the body's own attempt to stabilize the damaged joint. This type of arthritis can occur not only in your knees and hips, but also in your fingers, spine, and big toe. You could spot the damage on X-rays by the time you're 40, and you'll likely start showing gradual minor symptoms during the next decade or so.

Secondary osteoarthritis. A hard tackle in football, a broken bone, or damage caused by another type of arthritis

HOW RHEUMATOID ARTHRITIS DAMAGES THE JOINTS

Inflammation is a normal part of the immune system's effort to protect the body: As white blood cells—attracted to the site of an infected scrape, for example—attempt to destroy bacteria or other harmful foreign organisms, they produce a reaction that triggers inflammation. In other words, inflammation shows that the immune system is at work. In rheumatoid arthritis, this natural immune response goes awry and, for unknown reasons, begins attacking healthy tissues—first in the joints and, later on, possibly throughout the body.

In the first stages, white blood cells flock to the joint and release products that inflame the synovial membrane and cause fluid to accumulate within the joint. The joint becomes red, warm, swollen, and painful. In most people, the disease progresses no further, but in severe cases, an invasive mass of tissue begins to grow on the surface of the cartilage. It produces enzymes that eat away at the

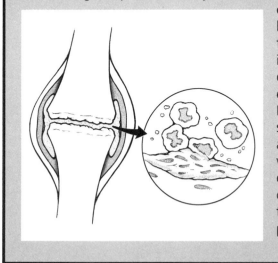

cartilage and bone. Without treatment, joint instability and deformity may eventually result. Fortunately, lifestyle measures and treatment with NSAIDs or other drugs can control symptoms in many people with RA.

can cause secondary osteoarthritis. Overuse, or doing the same motion repeatedly, can also cause it. In most cases normal activities don't produce osteoarthritis, however. It's all a matter of degree. Jogging, for example, when done for fun or exercise, is usually perfectly safe, but professional runners or marathoners can literally run into trouble. This, in a way, is like lots of small injuries happening all the time. If, for example, your job requires you to climb stairs frequently while carrying heavy loads, you're more likely to have osteoarthritis in your knees than people whose jobs are "on the level." If you play lots of tennis or operate a hand drill every day, you're a bit more likely to have osteoarthritis in your hand or wrist. Because secondary osteoarthritis involves extra stress on your joints, it can creep up at a younger age than primary osteoarthritis.

What about rheumatoid arthritis? Unfortunately, the causes aren't so clear. As mentioned, some researchers theorize that it's the body's reaction to a virus or a bacterium, but no one is sure if this is really true or what trigger might be involved.

Here is a general overview of the causes of major types of arthritis and related ailments. (All of these, and several others, are discussed in more detail in chapter 7.)

Bursitis. Excessive pressure on tissues around specific joints, such as kneeling or working a long time with your arms raised overhead.

Fibromyalgia. Unknown, but possibly linked to chemical changes in the body caused by prolonged high stress.

Gout. Too much uric acid. Your body may simply produce too much, or you may get it from eating too many foods that contain purines (substances that change to uric acid) or by drinking too much. (Alcohol contains purines, and it also keeps you from getting rid of purines in your urine.) The most common cause, however, is failure of your kidneys to secrete normal amounts of uric acid. There may be a genetic link.

Lupus. Unknown, but possible genetic, hormonal, or racial link.

Lyme disease. Bacteria from infected deer tick.

Polymyalgia rheumatica and giant cell arteritis. Unknown.

WHAT DOES TREATMENT INVOLVE?

For many lucky people, as we've noted earlier, osteo-arthritis may not progress much beyond morning stiffness and mild pain in the knees and hands. And for many others, very simple therapies or lifestyle changes will take care of the problem. For some, however, osteo-arthritis can sometimes become so painful that walking is almost impossible.

The good news is that much can be done to prevent such a dire outcome. Strategies as simple as exercise, improving your posture, or losing weight to ease the strain on your joints can help tremendously. Medication such as aspirin or injected corticosteroid can ease the pain or reduce swelling, and damaged cartilage can sometimes be trimmed or smoothed by a procedure called arthroscopy. And the pain may lessen as the roughened ends of your bones become "polished" through use over time.

In some cases, healthy cartilage can be grown in a test tube and then surgically "patched" into the joint. In an even more exciting development, researchers are currently testing substances that can help stimulate your body to grow new cartilage in your joint. And when all else fails, the damaged joint sometimes can be replaced with an artificial one, made of stainless steel and plastic. (Surgery options are discussed in chapter 8.)

Rheumatoid arthritis is trickier to treat. When you have flare-ups, you must rest the affected area so it won't deteriorate and the swelling can go down. But if you don't exercise at all or stretch or use your muscles and joints, gradually you'll become unable to use them—much like a vehicle that's been left rusting in the backyard. That's why your treatment should include a careful combination of rest and exercise to keep your limbs working, without making the trouble worse. This can be a delicate balancing act, which is why you need an excellent relationship with a good doctor and possibly the services of a good physical therapist as well.

During a flare-up, your doctor may advise you not only to rest but also to keep the painful joint completely still—either by lying flat or by using a splint to keep the joint from moving. Between flare-ups, it's usually a good idea to exercise, but do it cautiously, being sure to stop before your pain grows severe. Although exercise does help by keeping you fit and feeling better, it won't make the condition disappear. Various medications are also used to fight rheumatoid arthritis, including drugs that decrease inflammation, such as aspirin or steroids, gold salts, and antimalarial drugs. (You'll find these covered in chapter 6.) And, if need be, surgery can replace or repair damaged joints.

Other types of arthritis and related conditions respond to many of the same treatment methods, but some types, such as the arthritis of Lyme disease and arthritis caused by gonorrhea bacteria, require treatment with antibiotics. We'll discuss these diseases in depth in chapter 7.

CAN I PREVENT ARTHRITIS?

You cannot prevent most forms of this disease. But you certainly *can* reduce the risk of getting significant osteoarthritis—and slow its development if you already have it—primarily by controlling your weight. In one study, women who lost an average of 11 pounds reduced the development of osteoarthritis in their knees. And those overweight women who lost the most improved the most, reducing their pain and other symptoms by half. Although obviously extra weight can strain major weight-bearing joints, such as knees and hips, another study suggested that extra weight also encouraged osteoarthritis in other joints. Possibly, too much body fat directly affects our cartilage, making those extra pounds more of an enemy than we thought.

You can also help reduce your risk of early osteoarthritis by protecting yourself from injuries, say from competitive contact sports or repetitive motions. If you're a linebacker or wrestler by profession, there's not much you can do other than use protective padding and keep in tiptop shape. But the rest of us can take all reasonable precautions. We should always keep our muscles strong to help support our joints, and in sports we should warm up carefully, use proper equipment such as the right shoes, and follow a balanced exercise program that keeps the whole body in shape rather than just parts of it. (You'll find tips on exercise programs in chapter 10.) On the job and throughout the day, we can try to find ways to avoid nonstop repetitive motion, take breaks when possible, and, again, keep our muscles strong and limber.

Gout is triggered by high levels of uric acid, which comes from a substance called purines; people prone to gout can help protect themselves by limiting their intake of alcohol and foods high in purines. These include liver, kidneys, brains, and sweetbreads.

Lyme disease can be prevented only by avoiding tick bites and getting prompt treatment if bitten. And, as far as anyone knows so far, there is unfortunately no way to prevent rheumatoid arthritis. Some studies have indicated that sensitivity to certain foods can trigger rheumatoid arthritis attacks in a few people, but this is rare.

COPING WITH A CHRONIC CONDITION

"Chronic" is a technical-sounding word with a lot of personal impact. According to one dictionary definition, chronic means "constantly vexing, weakening, or troubling." If you have a chronic form of arthritis—most often that's an inflammatory type such as rheumatoid arthritis or lupus—it's the suggestion of *constant* in "chronic" that can wear you down. But the real picture is not as bleak as it sounds.

With chronic arthritis, you may find at first that what's hardest to deal with isn't the physical pain but rather the emotional consequences it can bring. You may fear that chronic means you'll never experience any relief. Like many others in your situation, you may find yourself struggling with thoughts like these:

- I'm falling apart.
- I'm going to lose control of my life.
- I'll lose my independence.
- I'll lose my appearance.
- I won't be able to work.
- I'll be in constant pain.

The fact is, however, that most of these fears are never realized. You may have a chronic condition that requires a new kind of awareness—and, yes, in that case it is something you will need to pay attention to for the rest of your life. But chronic doesn't have to mean constant; most types of chronic arthritis flare up now and then but don't cause relentless pain every day.

When you're hurting and searching for relief, it's easy to become discouraged. But hang in there. It's important to understand that because of the nature of chronic arthritis, medical treatment is based on a trial and error approach. So, although there are many effective medicines and treatments for pain, it takes time to find the combination that's effective for you. Your doctor may have to try you on several different drugs, for several months each, for example. And even though it's hard to wait for the most effective relief, this trial and error approach is proper treatment. Have faith in the process, and realize that though the wait may be frustrating, it will pay off in the end.

And many kinds of more immediate practical help are available. There are effective physical treatments for pain, therapists who can help you modify your home or workplace so maneuvering is easier, support groups so you'll know you're not alone, and abundant gadgets and gizmos and clever ideas to help you cope more easily. (You'll read more about these helps in chapter 9.)

In the great majority of cases, people with chronic arthritis continue to live enjoyable, fulfilling lives that may be modified in some ways but are no less meaningful. You can become resigned to the condition but never resign from life.

STRUGGLING WITH ARTHRITIS

You may be one of the many lucky people whose arthritis is a minor inconvenience, or you may have a kind such as bursitis that can be completely healed and then is gone for good. But for some of us, especially those with rheumatoid arthritis or other inflammatory types such as lupus, arthritis is more serious.

Most of us are used to simple diseases or health problems. You get a cold; it goes away in a week or so. You have a headache; you take an aspirin. You have an infection; you take an antibiotic. You break a bone; you wear a cast and the bone heals.

But unfortunately, arthritis is not so simple. Rheumatoid arthritis, in particular, will wax and wane, it will get better and get worse, all at unpredictable times. Many medications won't work instantly, and still others may not work for you at all or may have such uncomfortable side effects that you can't use them.

When you find out you have arthritis or a related disorder, you may feel that you're falling apart or that grimmer developments are just around the corner. Many people who discover they have arthritis become depressed: They think they're going to die or completely lose control of their lives. It's like being caught up, unarmed, in a war you didn't know existed, with battles erupting off and on and no armistice in sight. But if you work with your doctor and muster all the patience you can, you'll eventually find relief.

For many people, particularly the majority with osteoarthritis, the fear is greater than the problem itself. It may help to put your troubles in perspective: Think about a Rolls-Royce, a finely crafted piece of machinery. As a Rolls gets older, the shock absorbers may begin to squeak a bit after a certain number of miles and may need to be repaired or even replaced. But the car is still a Rolls-Royce, built to last. Similarly, your body is still a wonderful mechanism and will last with loving care—it has just developed a few squeaks and rattles.

WORKING WITH YOUR DOCTORS

Doctors, of course, understand the difficulties of dealing with arthritis. They know that now and then you may find yourself feeling frustrated or depressed or even tempted to stop taking your medications when they don't seem to be working. Or, if you forget that trial and error is the name of the arthritis treatment plan, you may lose faith in your doctor and wonder if she is doing her job properly.

What you need to keep in mind is that not everyone responds the same way to the same medicine. While a certain medicine may work for most people, it may not work for you and you may have to move on to another. This doesn't mean that either your doctor or the drug is a failure. It's just an unfortunate reminder that humans all respond differently. We are wonderful, intricate creations, and no two of us, including identical twins, are exactly alike. This makes life more interesting, but it also makes treatment of a disease such as rheumatoid arthritis more difficult.

What helps most is understanding that your doctor does have a plan and that each phase of treatment has an end point. So each time your doctor prescribes a medication, ask how long it will take before results may show up and how long he wants you to take this medication. Ask what signs to look for and what changes to expect. It may help if you keep a small notebook with you and jot down notes about your symptoms (or use a small tape recorder if writing is painful).

Always think of yourself as an active participant in your health care. You can help your doctor find the best treatment for your arthritis by carefully noting symptoms and changes and reporting them. You'll find that the frustrating process of finding the right treatment for you becomes a lot easier when you're involved in the decision making.

And be patient. Remind yourself that arthritis medications don't work overnight. Because of the nature of this disease and because of how different we all are from one another, the very medication that worked just fine for your neighbor may not be the right one for you.

And no matter what else you do, keep talking to your doctor. It's the best way to ensure that the two of you can forge a partnership in healing that will allow you to take charge of your disease—and your health.

CHAPTER 2

How to Tell if You Have Arthritis

You roll out of bed, but the minute your feet hit the floor you realize that your knees ache painfully. Or maybe everything hurts—arms, shoulders, legs, hips—and you feel so exhausted that all you want to do is curl back up in your cozy bed.

Are these just the normal aches and pains from too many sets of tennis, too many miles walking, or too many hours on your knees in the garden? Do you just need a rest and maybe an ice pack? Or could these be symptoms of arthritis?

There's no surefire way to tell if you have arthritis without visiting a doctor, but there are some basic clues to cue you when to suspect arthritis or a related condition— and when it's time to visit a doctor. It will help for you to become familiar with various symptoms, so you'll know what to watch for. Although accurate diagnosis involves several tests, your symptoms, no matter how apparently minor or unrelated, are valuable clues that will help your doctor decide which tests are appropriate.

In this chapter we'll discuss these symptoms, how to prepare effectively for a visit to the doctor, and the tests you may encounter.

WHEN DO YOU NEED TO SEE A DOCTOR?

Arthritis can have many symptoms, and you cannot diagnose it on your own. But any of these warning signs may suggest arthritis:

+ You feel stiff after you get up.
+ One of your joints won't move normally.
+ A joint is red or warm to the touch.
+ You've lost weight and have fever and joint pain.
+ One or more joints are swollen.

If you have one of more of these symptoms for longer than two weeks, it's time to make a doctor's appointment and be checked for arthritis. (If you have muscle or joint pain for more than two weeks *without* other symptoms, it's still a good idea to see a doctor. You may not have arthritis, but you may have something else that needs treatment, such as a bone or nerve problem.)

And be aware that some joint problems are caused by infection from a virus, bacterium, or fungus that spreads through the bloodstream. So if you feel weak and have chills or a fever, in addition to feeling pain and stiffness in a joint that's red or warm to the touch, immediately head for the doctor's office or the emergency room if it's after hours. These can be symptoms of infectious arthritis that requires prompt treatment with antibiotics.

HOW WILL ARTHRITIS MAKE YOU FEEL?

All arthritis involves aches and pains. But where it hurts, when, and how much are frequently determined by the type you have.

Osteoarthritis. Symptoms of osteoarthritis often come on gradually. You may start to notice stiffness in your joints when you first get up in the morning. You may have a joint you hurt in an accident or fall that aches a bit just before a rainstorm. Your knee may hurt every time you bend it. You may experience swelling around certain joints and find that they are less flexible than before. Or small lumps may develop on the joints of your fingers.

These symptoms usually begin to pop up when you're in your 40s or 50s, but they can occur earlier. You may be a bit stiff in the morning, but you loosen up after 15 minutes or so. Later, you may feel some mild pain when you move your knee or finger or whichever joint is affected. When you do more of an activity that uses the affected joint, you hurt more. When you rest, you hurt less.

For some people, that's it: They will never have any more complex or painful symptoms. They'll pop an occasional aspirin or ibuprofen tablet, take a few more rest days than when they were younger, and just get on with life. In others, however, the cartilage breaks down so much that bone is practically rubbing against bone, and using the joint is so excruciating that it's next to impossible. Painful bone spurs can develop at the ends of the bones.

Joints that crackle when moved may also be a sign of arthritis, and sometimes our finger joints may become enlarged. (When this happens to the end finger joint, the swellings are called Heberden's nodes; when it happens to the middle joints, they're called Bouchard's nodes.)

Rheumatoid arthritis. If you have rheumatoid arthritis, initially you may ache or be stiff, particularly in the morning or after sitting still for periods of time. This discomfort is caused by swelling in the joint lining. Morning stiffness tends to last longer than with osteoarthritis—up to an hour, until your regular medication kicks in. Your joints may also be painful, swollen, and warm to the touch, although this will come and go. You'll likely feel fatigued, and you may run a low fever, not feel much like eating, and develop anemia. Small lumps called nodules may show up, particularly in your elbows if you tend to lean them for long periods on a table or desk. Rheumatoid arthritis can disappear for a time—this is called remission—but in some people it can also deform joints so much that doing the common tasks of day-to-day life is a real challenge.

Related conditions. Other types of arthritis and related diseases, such as gout, lupus, and Lyme disease, may have similar symptoms. (Later, in chapter 7, we'll discuss these conditions in more detail, along with a few less common ones.) For now, here's a rundown of the basic symptoms.

- **Bursitis.** Dull pain in or around a joint that gets worse when you move.
- **Fibromyalgia.** Total body pain, or pain in the muscles, ligaments, and tendons, and fatigue.
- **Gout.** Sudden painful attacks, often in the big toe, and often beginning at night.
- **Lupus.** Joint and muscle aches; warm, swollen joints; fatigue; usually rashes. Often fever, sometimes chest pain when you breathe.
- **Lyme disease.** Sometimes a round rash with a clear center, with early symptoms similar to those of the flu. Later symptoms include muscle aches, joint pain, and fatigue.
- **Polymyalgia rheumatica.** Aches and stiffness in the neck, shoulders, and hips, worse after not moving; most often in women older than 50.

How Your Doctor Diagnoses Arthritis

As we discussed in chapter 1, your doctor has two ways of making a diagnosis of arthritis: by determining the pattern (number and location) of joints involved and by determining whether other parts of the body are also affected. He'll also want to be sure to distinguish between arthritis and bursitis, a painful inflammation of the fluid-filled sacs around your joints that allow muscles, tendons, ligaments, and skin to slide over each other. Bursitis requires a different kind of examination and treatment, which we'll take a look at shortly.

To diagnose the two major kinds of arthritis, osteoarthritis and rheumatoid arthritis, your doctor will ask you many questions and possibly have you fill out a questionnaire about your activity level, general health, family history, and smoking or drinking habits. He'll examine your joints, checking for pain, stiffness, and limited range of motion. Your doctor will also look for joint deformities and other physical signs such as small lumps on your joints, rashes, and an enlarged spleen. And he'll check for specifics that may indicate one type of arthritis or another.

Osteoarthritis. An examination of the joints of your hands, arms, legs, and feet will tell your doctor which joints are affected and whether they are affected on both sides of your body. Usually, in osteoarthritis, you'll first be affected on one side. Your doctor will also examine the joints of your spine.

Osteoarthritis usually does not occur in the wrist but, as we've mentioned, you may have small lumps on your finger joints, called Heberden's nodes (on the end joint) and Bouchard's nodes (on the middle joint). Your joints should feel cool, not warm, to the touch.

If your doctor strongly suspects osteoarthritis after the examination, he may order X-rays to check for bone and cartilage damage. Diagnostic tests may include taking synovial fluid from swollen joints to check for an elevated white blood cell count or bacteria that could mean an infection or for crystals that indicate gout or another disorder. And a "sed rate" blood test (also called erythrocyte sedimentation rate, or ESR) will also be done to measure

THE HEAVY ARTILLERY

Sometimes your doctor will prescribe special tests to check for bone or tissue damage or abnormalities. Generally these tests are expensive and time-consuming, so they aren't used unless specifically required.

CT scan. The full name for this is computerized axial tomography, and it's also called a CAT scan. In this test, a very thin X-ray passes through your body. Because bone and fluid absorb different amounts of radiation, they show up very differently on the scan. For better visibility, sometimes dye is injected into a vein. A CAT scan shows internal tissues much better than a standard X-ray and also does a better job of revealing arthritis around the spinal cord. For this procedure, you lie flat on a special table while the X-rays pass through you.

MRI. This is short for magnetic resonance imaging, and it can let the doctor see erosion that doesn't appear on X-rays. The major value of MRI, which involves no radiation, is that it can show early changes in bone and abnormalities of the soft tissues around the bone. MRI can show if your knee cartilage is torn, for example, but standard X-rays cannot. Here's how it works: Because the hydrogen in our bodies responds to the magnetic field, areas where we have the most water (made up of hydrogen and oxygen) respond differently than areas with less water. The resultant image will show up abnormalities. During an MRI, you lie on a special table that is moved into a narrow tube that may make you feel as if you're in a science fiction movie. In the tube, a strong magnetic field is passed over your body, and you have to lie quite still. You may begin to feel a little claustrophobic, but it helps to concentrate on breathing smoothly and evenly and picturing a peaceful scene in your mind, such as floating in water at the beach. The procedure is noisy but painless, and your visualizations will help you stay relaxed.

the amount of inflammation in your body. Generally, your
sed rate is not likely to be elevated if you have osteoarthritis.

Rheumatoid arthritis. The pain or other symptoms
you describe to your doctor give important clues for diagnosis. Other signs are red, swollen, warm joints; misshapen
fingers; or small nodules under the skin (one in five people
with rheumatoid arthritis will have these nodules). In the
early stages, rheumatoid arthritis can be quite difficult to
diagnose. In most people, however, a blood test will ultimately show elevated rheumatoid factor. In the first few
months of rheumatoid arthritis, this test may be negative,
but in 8 out of 10 people with arthritis, it will eventually
be positive. The amount of rheumatoid factor increases as
the disease progresses. But to complicate matters, unfortunately, it can also be high in people who don't have
rheumatoid arthritis.

Along with the rheumatoid factor test, your doctor will
probably run tests for sed rate, red blood cell count, and
possibly other measurements. He may also withdraw fluid
from your painful joints to check for infection and inflammation. If you have rheumatoid arthritis, you may have a
high sed rate and mild anemia.

And if you've had rheumatoid arthritis for at least six
months, X-rays may show damage to your cartilage and
bones. Because cartilage has deteriorated and the bone
has eroded, the space between cartilage and bone where
the deterioration has occurred will be apparent.

Other less common symptoms of rheumatoid arthritis
don't show up in the joints. These include anemia, dry eyes,
dry mouth and other dry membranes, inflamed eye tissues,
and carpal tunnel syndrome. More serious but fortunately
less common symptoms are inflammation of the membrane
over the heart (pericarditis), inflammation of the membranes
around the lungs (pleurisy), and rarely, Felty's syndrome (a

combination of conditions that includes low white blood cell count and an enlarged spleen). For more on complications, see "Rheumatoid Arthritis and *Other* Body Parts," on page 32.

A LOOK AT OTHER TYPES OF ARTHRITIS

Here is an overview of the *symptoms* and *tests* your doctor will evaluate to find out if you have another type of arthritis or a related disease. (You'll find detailed discussions of these ailments in chapter 7.)

Bursitis

Symptoms: Dull pain that increases with movement and may awaken you at night. The pain is likely to begin more abruptly than arthritis pain. The area around the joint may be swollen and warm when you touch it; if the bursa is infected, the area around it will be red.

Tests: Your doctor may want to take X-rays to rule out other problems such as bone or cartilage damage that could be causing inflammation in nearby tissues. Although bursae are usually inflamed from overuse, bursitis also can be caused by infection, so your doctor may want to remove fluid from the bursa to test it for infection by measuring the white blood cell count and checking for bacterial growth.

Fibromyalgia

Symptoms: Pain in the muscles, ligaments, and tendons. Another is fatigue, even after a full night's sleep, and some people may have occasional numbness or tingling, headaches, and gastrointestinal problems. Also, women may suffer pain during menstruation.

Tests: Diagnosis involves eliminating other ailments, as fibromyalgia doesn't show up in X-rays or blood tests (but your doctor may want to do blood tests to check for arthritis or other diseases). The guidelines for diagnosis developed by the American College of Rheumatology in 1990 include having pain on both sides of your body for at least a three-month period, and feeling distinct pain in at least 11 of 18 trigger points when your doctor applies about nine pounds of pressure.

Gout

Symptoms: These extremely painful attacks come suddenly, often at night, in a matter of hours. Three times out of four, the pain is in the big toe, which becomes swollen, hot, and red. The pain is so extreme that often you can't even tolerate the pressure of a sheet draped over the foot. The pain gradually goes away after a week or two.

Tests: Your doctor will likely run blood tests checking your uric acid, sed rate, and white blood cell count. Most people with gout will have elevated blood uric acid levels—greater than 7 milligrams per deciliter (or dL) in men and 6 milligrams/dL in women. During an attack your sed rate and white blood cell count will also be high. If your doctor withdraws synovial fluid from a joint, uric acid crystals will be present.

Lupus

Symptoms: Joint and muscle aches and warm, swollen joints. You may also be tired, have a low fever, lose your appetite, lose weight, and have rashes and mouth ulcers.

Tests: Blood tests to find specific antibodies. These may include FANA, anti-DNA, and anti-Sm, but because other conditions can give positive test results, a blood test alone isn't a definite diagnosis.

Lyme disease

Symptoms: You may see a circular rash around the tick bite. Two-thirds of the people infected have an expanding red ring with a clear center, but it's easy to overlook. (As the infecting tiny tick is smaller than a pinhead, about half of people with Lyme can't recall having been bitten.) Next you'll have flu-like symptoms: chills, fever, headaches, a stiff

RHEUMATOID ARTHRITIS
AND *OTHER* BODY PARTS

Rheumatoid arthritis affects your joints, of course, but it can also cause trouble in other parts of your body. Most such complications are uncommon, however. If you have any symptoms of these problems, report them promptly to your doctor.

Anemia. If you are weak, pale, and short of breath, you may have anemia, which is caused by a low red blood cell count. Anemia can be caused by rheumatoid arthritis or by use of nonsteroidal anti-inflammatory drugs (or NSAIDs) that cause stomach bleeding. As many as two-thirds of people with rheumatoid arthritis may become anemic.

Felty's syndrome. A cluster of symptoms including anemia, an enlarged spleen, and a low white blood cell count is called Felty's syndrome, an extremely rare complication of rheumatoid arthritis. The low white blood cell count may lead to infection. This unusual syndrome can also cause sores or dark patches on your skin.

Neuropathy. When inflamed joints put pressure on nearby nerves or when the blood supply is restricted by vasculitis (see next page), nerve damage, or neuropathy, may result. It can cause numbness, tingling, or weakness. Carpal

neck, swollen lymph nodes, fatigue, muscle aches, and joint pain. Initially, the arthritis of Lyme disease is migratory, or travels from joint to joint. Later, Lyme causes monarthritis, or arthritis of one joint, which is almost always the knee. If untreated, the disease can include late symptoms of severe headache and fatigue, drooping of face muscles, and pain or numbness.

Tests: Lyme disease has typically been diagnosed with a blood test called the Lyme titer, which shows the presence tunnel syndrome, for example, is neuropathy of the thumb and middle three fingers.

Pericarditis. This is an inflammation of the membrane that covers the heart, called the pericardium. It may cause discomfort in your chest or make it difficult for you to breathe.

Pleurisy. When the linings of the lungs are inflamed, the condition is called pleurisy. Like pericarditis, it can cause chest discomfort or trouble breathing.

Rheumatoid nodules. These inflammatory cells collect under the skin near joints and are generally harmless. They can also occur in your lung, heart, or eyes, but even then they usually don't cause damage.

Scleritis and episcleritis. Inflammation of the outer layers of the eye causes these problems. Your eyes may become painful and red, and your vision may change. Either condition requires visits to the ophthalmologist.

Sjögren's syndrome. Sometimes along with arthritis, you'll find your mouth feels dry and your eyes do, too. These symptoms may indicate Sjögren's syndrome. (You'll read more about it in chapter 7.)

Vasculitis. This is inflammation of the blood vessels, and it can limit your blood flow. Symptoms can include sores on the skin or problems with your fingernails.

of Lyme bacteria antibodies, called spirochetes, after the first symptoms appear. A new antibody test, however, can be used for diagnosis when Lyme disease is suspected, long before arthritis and other symptoms arrive.

Polymyalgia rheumatica (PMR)

Symptoms: Aches and stiffness in the neck, shoulders, and hips in a person over age 50 and often closer to 70. As is true of virtually all forms of arthritis, pain is generally worse in the morning or after resting. What's destructive about PMR is the severity and broad distribution of the pain, which can occur over the muscles and joints of the neck, both shoulder areas, and the areas of the hips. PMR is also associated with other symptoms, including low fever, fatigue, weight gain, lethargy (also called malaise), and joint swelling.

Tests: Blood tests for anemia and systemic inflammation. Usually sed rate is more than 40 millimeters per hour, and rheumatoid factor and FANA tests are negative. Sometimes diagnosis is made only after a "test" dose of corticosteroids: If you do not respond dramatically, your doctor can be sure you do not have polymyalgia rheumatica. Your platelet count may also be high.

HOW TO PREPARE FOR YOUR DOCTOR VISIT

The best way to prepare is to take time to think about your goals before your appointment. Basically, they involve both *getting* the information you need to use your treatment most effectively and *giving* the information your doctor needs to design the best treatment plan. Start by going in with a small pad and pen or a miniature tape recorder to take notes. Here are more tips to help you make the most of your time with your doctor.

List your medications. It's important for your doctor to know what medicines you take—whether they are taken occasionally or every day, are prescribed, or over-the-counter. Make a list of *all* the pills you take, including vitamins, aspirin, and any other remedies or pills you buy without a prescription.

Be ready to describe your symptoms. Your doctor will want to know when the pain started, what type of pain it is, and what makes it worse. Good descriptive words are "sharp," "stabbing," "dull" or "achy," and "throbbing." You'll

find it easier to jot these down before you visit the doctor.
Your doctor may ask questions such as:

- When did your pain start?
- How long does it last?
- How much does it hurt, say on a scale of 1 to 10?
- Do you have trouble getting out of a chair?
- Do you have trouble getting in and out of a car?
- Have you stopped or cut back any activities because of this pain?
- Which joints hurt?
- What causes the pain or makes it worse?
- When during the day do you feel the pain?
- What time of day does it hurt the worst?
- Does anything relieve the pain?
- Have your joints been red or swollen?
- Are you stiff in the morning?
- Does anyone in your family have arthritis? What kind?
- Have you ever had an accident or injured this joint?
- How are you sleeping?
- How has this affected your life?

Describe your daily lifestyle. Because so many joint
problems are caused or made worse by certain activities,
your doctor will want to know details about what you do
at work and what types of things you do during the day.
Just about everything can be relevant here: gardening, golf-
ing, how long you spend at a computer keyboard, how you
sleep at night. Jot down notes so that you'll remember to
mention things.

CHAPTER 3

Finding Medical Care

Every morning for the past two weeks you've awakened with aching joints. Or your hip has made you so miserable that you couldn't help snapping at your spouse. Or your fingers hurt so much it's difficult to grip a pen to do your favorite crossword puzzle.

You know something is wrong. You're wondering if you have arthritis. But you're not sure if you need to see a doctor. Arthritis is just the price of getting older, right? And what can doctors do about it, anyway?

Plenty. And doctors and other health care professionals can also help you learn to help yourself. In this chapter, we'll tell you how to find the best possible care and what a wide range of support is available.

WHY YOU SHOULDN'T WAIT IT OUT

Only a doctor can tell you if your knee hurts because of arthritis or because you tripped over the cat last week. She is also the only person who can tell you what sort of arthritis you have. And that's an important distinction, because treatments for the two most common types—osteoarthritis and rheumatoid arthritis—are very different.

Rheumatoid arthritis, as well as other inflammatory diseases, involves severe inflammation that, if left untreated, can seriously damage your joints and lead to complications elsewhere in the body such as in the heart and lungs.

Doctors now believe that beginning treatment early is vital because much irreversible joint damage occurs in the first two years after the disease hits. It's harsh but true—early intervention with rheumatoid arthritis can mean the difference in whether or not it will cripple you.

It isn't as crucial to rush to the doctor with osteoarthritis, as the damage it does happens more slowly and is not as devastating. But a doctor can help you learn to avoid activities or motions that damage your cartilage or aggravate your condition. Sometimes damaged cartilage can be surgically trimmed, and in a few cases it can be "patched." And treatments just around the corner, which some doctors are already recommending, may slow cartilage damage. Regardless of what treatment is needed, *early* medical attention can prevent joints from "freezing up" or losing mobility. Because if your joint hurts, you'll tend to move it only to the point that it begins to pain you—and eventually you might become unable to move it any farther.

WHOM DO YOU NEED TO SEE?

The best place to start is usually with a visit to your family doctor or internist, who can run tests and either make a diagnosis or decide that you need more specialized care. In some cases, your own doctor will be able to guide you in your fight against arthritis; in others you may need the services of a rheumatology specialist. It all depends on the qualifications and inclinations of your doctor, what type of arthritis you have, and how advanced it is. Here's how to figure out who can help you best.

Family practitioner (FP) or general internist. Most family doctors are family practitioners or internists. A family practitioner takes care of children and adults; an internist is a specialist for adults. The advantage of your internist or FP is that he knows the whole "you." This can be especially helpful if you have other ongoing ailments, such as diabetes, high blood pressure, or asthma. Depending on your condition, some FPs or internists can treat your arthritis on their own; others will work with a specialist called a rheumatologist to whom they refer you; still others may turn your arthritis care over completely to a rheumatologist so you'll get all the expertise you need.

Primary care physician. This is just another name for the person who provides most of your medical care: your family doctor or practitioner, a GP (general practitioner), or an internist. This doctor can refer you to more specialized care if needed.

Rheumatologist. A rheumatologist is an internist who has had an additional two or three years of training in arthritis and specializes in treating rheumatic diseases and more complicated forms of arthritis. A rheumatologist is expert at diagnosing and can run and interpret complicated tests. He can also develop treatment plans and provide ongoing care. (Bear in mind that if you have only mild or moderate osteoarthritis, however, you probably don't need a rheumatologist.)

SPECIALISTS YOU MAY ENCOUNTER

Your doctor may refer you to other specialists, depending on your health needs. These can include the following.

Ophthalmologist. An ophthalmologist provides eye care and treatment. Some types of arthritis, such as Sjögren's syndrome and juvenile rheumatoid arthritis, may cause eye problems that can damage vision if not treated, such as dry eyes or inflammation of the eyes (scleritis and episcleritis).

Physiatrist. A physiatrist specializes in helping people with muscle, bone, or nervous system problems, using treatments such as exercise therapy, heat and ice, electrical stimulation, and ultrasound. A physiatrist can prescribe medication but concentrates on nondrug treatments.

Neurologist. This doctor specializes in muscles and nerves and assesses nerve damage.

Neurosurgeon. This type of surgeon operates on the back, neck, and brain. (But it's unlikely you'd need brain surgery for arthritis, of course.)

Orthopedic surgeon. Surgery such as arthroscopy or joint replacement is done by an orthopedic surgeon, who specializes in bone, muscle, and joint problems. Also called an orthopedist, this doctor can prescribe other treatments for arthritis, including prescription medication, physical therapy, or braces or splints. An orthopedist can diagnose problems as well as provide ongoing care.

OTHER HEALTH CARE PROFESSIONALS WHO CAN HELP YOU

Doctors today emphasize whole-body arthritis treatment that includes physical therapy, an exercise program, diet where appropriate, various devices to support and relieve your joints, and training you to move and work in a way that spares your joints. It's a team approach to everything that affects your arthritis: what you eat, how you move, your medication, and even your emotional state.

Here are some of the professionals who may be on your team.

Physical therapist. This therapist has a bachelor's degree or graduate degree in physical therapy and is trained to help relieve your pain without using drugs. Treatment may include exercises to strengthen your muscles or improve your joints' range of motion (how far you can move them), endurance exercise, water therapy, hot or cold treatments, ultrasound, and relaxation techniques. Physical therapists can also teach you how to help yourself; they can assess you, your condition, and your lifestyle and prescribe an individualized exercise program. They can also advise you on body mechanics, such as showing you ways to sit or stand that stress your joints less, and they can help you learn to use crutches and canes if needed. (You'll find more on physical therapists in chapter 4.)

Occupational therapist. It may not sound like fun to have someone come into your home and show you new ways of doing things—maybe even suggesting that you move your furniture! But after you've tried an occupational therapist's suggestions, you'll be happy you did. An occupational therapist focuses on ways to make your day-to-day tasks much easier—both at home and at work. This includes new or slightly different ways to get out of bed, rise from a chair, dress, eat, and work so that you feel less pain or can do more than you thought you could manage. Occupational therapists can particularly help people with rheumatoid arthritis or other inflammatory diseases learn how and when to use splints and other helpful devices. Their job is to evaluate your home or office, suggest rearranging things for less joint stress, and offer you energy-saving ideas. These may be as simple as storing related items together in your kitchen so that you don't have to open cabinets and move as many things when you cook.

Podiatrist. This foot specialist can recommend types of footwear that will help relieve pain. Podiatrists can fit you with custom-made orthotics (a device that goes inside your shoes to ease strain or make them fit better) and can prescribe anti-inflammatories.

Nutritionist. It's not easy to change your diet or plan meals to meet all of your nutritional needs. A nutritionist will advise you on your food choices, help you learn ways to lose weight if needed, or devise a personalized eating plan. Many are registered dietitians, certified by the American Dietetic Association.

Registered nurse. RNs can often answer your day-to-day questions or check with the doctor for you when you have a question or problem between office visits.

In addition to medical specialists, you may want to see one or both of the following.

Exercise instructor. This can include the water aerobics instructor at the Y, a beginner's exercise teacher, or the friendly weight-training coach at your local health club. Many classes are specially designated for senior citizens or people with arthritis, and they can be very helpful. Because the training of instructors varies greatly, it's a good idea to first ask what experience the instructor has in working with people with arthritis or joint problems. And you should, of course, clear any exercise program before you start with your doctor or physical therapist, who can offer advice on when to ease up and how to protect your joints during exercises. He can also tell you which movements or exercises might aggravate your condition rather than help it.

Social worker. Arthritis can change your life, and these changes can be tough to deal with. This disease can be difficult both financially and emotionally, and social workers can give you real support. They can help you get job counseling or training, find out what benefits you are eligible for, and may be able to help you cope with the emotional pressures as well. (See box, "Dealing with Depression," for information on locating a social worker or therapist.)

EFFECTIVE COMMUNICATION WITH YOUR HEALTH CARE PROFESSIONAL

As we discussed in chapter 2, preparing ahead of time for your visit to the doctor is an important part of your arthritis treatment plan. Your list of the questions you need to ask, the medicines you're taking, and the details of how you're feeling will all help your doctor to improve the care you receive.

Once you're in the office, here's how you can communicate most effectively.

Establish your agenda early. If there's a major question or problem on your mind, be sure to let the doctor know early in your conversation. Say, for example, "I want to ask you about exercise today," so your doctor can pace himself and have time to give you all the information you need. (If you're almost out the door and add, "Oh, the major problem is . . . ," it'll be harder for him to help you.)

Offer clear details. You can pack a lot of information into a few words if you choose the right ones. Be as specific as you can. "I haven't been feeling well" doesn't tell your doctor much, but "I'm groggy in the mornings, but I don't have any trouble sleeping" gives clear, specific information that can help your doctor figure out what's going on. If you're describing pain, it helps to express the pain in terms of what you can and can't do. Instead of saying only "My hands hurt," give your doctor an example of just how the pain affects you, as in "My fingers hurt so much I can't hold a pen." That helps your doctor to understand much more clearly what's going on with you.

Don't be afraid to call. While you don't want to be on the phone to your doctor's office constantly, neither should you sit at home worrying whether a symptom is serious enough to report. If you have a troublesome symptom—a lump, a strong reaction to a medication, a severe pain—call your doctor's office. Be very clear: "I have been nauseated for three days and wonder if I should discontinue my medication or make an appointment." The nurse or receptionist will write your question down, relay it to the doctor, and call you back. It's quick, easy, and painless.

DEALING WITH DEPRESSION

Arthritis and its effects on your body—and sometimes side effects from your medication—can be tough to handle. You may feel overwhelmed at first by the immediate challenges of diagnosis and the search for the right pain relief. Sometimes it's hard to keep in mind that with treatment you're soon going to be feeling much better. Young people in particular can be devastated by the changes that diseases such as lupus, fibromyalgia, and Lyme disease can bring.

It's very common to feel down in the dumps when you discover you have arthritis. But there's no reason to be disabled by depression. Talk to your doctor. The great majority of depressed patients are treated very successfully by their internists or family physicians. Your doctor can help to determine whether yours is a normal reaction to the difficulties of coping with arthritis or whether you've developed a true clinical depression. Remember, too, that certain drugs can trigger depression. It's possible that a change in your medication will help your mood to rise. Also, your doctor can often ease your mental pain by changing how he treats the physical pain of your arthritis. If your body hurts less, chances are your mind will, too.

Finally, take note of what you're thinking and how often you're thinking it. Do you have a running monologue of hopeless-sounding comments going through your head? If, despite your best efforts to change them, your feelings of depression are persistent and severe, your doctor may either prescribe antidepressant medication, refer you to a therapist, or do both.

Your doctor or a friend may have an excellent therapist or counselor to recommend, and some states have referral organizations. Before starting therapy, however, be sure to give your insurance company a call to discover what types of therapists or counselors are covered.

Know when to fold 'em. You have every right to have a doctor you trust and can talk with. It's fine to change doctors if you feel you've reached an impasse, but you don't want to move on without first voicing your concerns. If you're feeling unhappy about your communication with your doctor, ask yourself: "Have I really talked straight enough so that my doctor knows what I'm upset about?" Give your doctor a chance to hear you out and try to fix the problem. Otherwise, you could find yourself in a new doctor's office and still feeling unsatisfied.

HOW *NOT* TO GET THE MOST OUT OF YOUR DOCTOR

As in any human relationship, what you get out of your visits with your doctor usually depends on what you put into them. Here are a few attitudes that just about guarantee that you'll shortchange yourself.

"Whatever you say." Some people look on their doctors as all-knowing, all-powerful beings and expect doctors simply to "fix" them. They want pills that will make them well, period. They don't want to be involved in their own health care, and they don't volunteer much information unless asked. They do exactly what the doctor says without asking questions or letting her know when things don't seem to be working or when they're feeling worse.

"Oh, *sure*." Some folks sit quietly while visiting a health care professional, but inside they're fuming or saying to themselves, "I'm not going to do what she says" or "This guy doesn't understand what I'm talking about." They go home and completely ignore the nutritionist's advice or don't fill the prescription the doctor has written. If this is you, you're essentially shooting yourself in the foot. You're not only wasting the money you're spending to visit a professional—and wasting the doctor's time as well—but also are likely hampering your progress in fighting the disease.

"I know what treatment I need." While it's great to learn all you can about your disease—and a good doctor welcomes your input—it's important to realize that some of what you read may not tell the whole story. Going to see your health care professional positive that you know what is best, perhaps waving a magazine article that promises a cure for your ailment, doesn't help. Instead, show your doctor the book or article and ask questions such as "What about treatment *xyz* I just read about?" Realize that a good doctor usually prefers to wait until not just one or two but *multiple* studies (on large groups of people, not just a few) have indicated consistent results and testing has shown that the proposed treatment is safe for you. And any new medicines, of course, must wait for approval from the Food and Drug Administration (FDA). The FDA testing process, while lengthy, assures you of quality and protects you from potentially serious complications that may not have shown up in a few limited or poorly designed studies.

CHAPTER 4

Fighting Arthritis
without Drugs

Some of the multiple forms of arthritis certainly won't cause you major problems. With moderate treatment and a few lifestyle changes you can often be up and about your business with little difficulty. Just as with many other common health problems, you take your medicine, or change your diet, or follow an exercise routine, and you get well.

But some kinds of arthritis, especially the inflammatory types like rheumatoid arthritis, don't follow this easygoing profile. As we've discussed, because every person is different, treatment that works well for one may not work for another. There's often no quick fix. Rheumatoid arthritis generally requires varying medications, and few of them work immediately. Osteoarthritis, too, may require a certain amount of trial and error to find what medication works and what doesn't. It can be a frustrating wait.

Fortunately, there are many effective ways to get a head start on your arthritis care and boost the effectiveness of your treatment without using medicine. Many of these methods are do-it-yourself techniques, and your active involvement makes all the difference. Here's a look at non-drug treatments that can give you powerful relief—and advice on a few that will just relieve you of your hard-earned dollars.

EDUCATE YOURSELF—AND OTHERS

Although it may not sound much like a treatment, learning about your disease is one of the best things you can do in the battle against arthritis. If you understand what's happening in your body and how treatment is likely to progress, not only can you participate in the healing process, but your condition won't seem so overwhelming.

Your family, too, will benefit from learning about arthritis. You may need to explain to your grandchildren, for instance, why you can't play with them some days but will be ready for a raincheck. Your children may be as worried as you are about your arthritis, and knowing the facts will help calm them. Your spouse will feel better if you can explain what types of things you can and can't do—why you may no longer want to vacuum daily or mow the lawn weekly, what effects your medications might have on you, or even why making love feels like a lot more fun in certain positions.

Your doctor is a good source of information about coping with the frustrations of arthritis. He can furnish brochures, refer you to other sources, and help you locate classes or presentations on arthritis and support groups. And there's a huge national organization out there—The Arthritis Foundation—whose primary purpose is to help, inform, and support people with arthritis. Contact your local chapter for some of its excellent educational materials.

HOT AND COLD TREATMENTS

Warmth can relieve pain by relaxing muscles, and cold can soothe pain and help reduce inflammation. And you can easily use them in ingenious ways to ease your pain.

- ◆ Soak in a warm tub or take a warm shower. If you have a huge hot tub, where you can submerge up to your chin in blissfully warm water, that's perfect. If not, a standard tub will do. If you don't have time to take a full bath and just your feet or hands are hurting, then soak them in a pan or bucket of warm water.

* To ease morning stiffness, turn on an electric blanket or electric mattress pad and enjoy the heat for a while before you get out of bed.
* Warm your clothes in the dryer for a few minutes before putting them on. This is especially comforting on chilly winter days.
* Use a warm compress on your painful joint, made of a towel soaked in hot water and wrung out. Or try an old-fashioned hot water bottle, placing a towel between it and your skin. (Don't leave either on for more than 20 minutes.)
* Use a heat lamp, but be careful to read directions and follow them closely.

Some health care professionals don't recommend heating pads, because if you happen to doze off you can burn yourself badly. If you do use one, however, place a kitchen timer with a loud ringer nearby with the timer set for 15 minutes.

Ice is also an excellent way to relieve pain and help fight minor inflammation, especially right after you have been active. There are several ways to apply ice. You can use any of the following:

* A cold pack that you store in the freezer
* An ice bag that you fill with ice
* A bag of crushed ice wrapped in a towel
* A bag of small frozen vegetables such as peas (and then have them for dinner)

As with hot treatments, leave the ice on no more than 20 minutes at a time, and be careful not to put it directly on your skin. You can wrap it in a towel, or put it in an ice bag you can buy at the drugstore. If you need to cool your ankles, feet, or hands, a bucket or dishpan with ice cubes and water is simple and effective. Just immerse and relax.

Physical therapists often use both hot and cold treatments. Hydrotherapy, supervised by a physical therapist, is done in a heated pool or whirlpool. While in the warm water, you may do gentle exercises aimed at improving your range of motion (how far you can move each joint), coordination, and circulation. Because the heat helps relieve pain and the water bears much of your weight, you'll be surprised by your ability to do exercises in the water that would be nearly impossible on dry land.

EXERCISE: FEELING BETTER IN A FITTER BODY

Exercise can be a very helpful tool in your arthritis care plan. If you're not already active, it can be both physically and mentally challenging to get going in a regular program, but the benefits can be a boon.

It's important to consult with your doctor before you start an exercise program, however. One of the most difficult things to master is the delicate balancing act between exercising enough to help yourself and exercising without hurting yourself. Your doctor can help you determine what kind of exercise will work best for you and when to use it, depending on what type of arthritis you have. (Remember, with over 100 forms, what helps one may aggravate another.) For example, the best way to make sure your gout won't go away is to shoot a few hoops while your foot hurts. And, if you're going through an episode of acute inflammation, such as from rheumatoid arthritis, exercise can harm you. But if things have cleared up and your doctor's given the green light, you can start creating a fitter body. And that should make you feel better all over.

The purpose of exercise is to keep joints moving, keep muscles strong, and build up your endurance. Because swollen joints can be worse when the pressure of your weight is put on them, at first the best exercises may be range-of-motion, moving each joint gently as far as you can, and simple moves such as straight leg raises. Exercising in water is wonderful because it supports your weight, which means you can move more without overtaxing your joints. A general rule: If, an hour after the exercise, you feel more pain than you did *before*, you're hindering more than helping. Stop that particular exercise.

Here are some basic tips:

+ During flare-ups of inflammatory diseases, don't work your joints. (You should, however, go through gentle range-of-motion exercises once or twice daily.)
+ Start slowly.
+ Relax your muscles with a gentle massage or warm bath or shower before workouts.
+ Warm up before working out by stretching gently and exercising slowly for 5 to 10 minutes and then stretching gently.
+ Be consistent; keep a regular exercise routine. You won't help yourself if you exercise every other day for a month and then stop for two weeks.
+ If your joints are inflamed or painful, stop.
+ Move slowly and steadily; never jerk or bounce.
+ Wear comfortable clothing and good exercise shoes.
+ Cool down by slowing the pace of your activity for the last 5 or 10 minutes, and then do some more gentle stretches.

There are three general types of exercise, and they all can be very helpful in an arthritis workout plan.

Range-of-motion. Each of our body parts is designed with a certain range of motion: You can normally reach or bend or twist a certain amount. But one of the biggest problems with arthritis is that because it hurts, we don't

EXERCISES TO IMPROVE RANGE OF MOTION IN ARTHRITIC JOINTS

Wrist flex. Place your arm on the edge of a table or on an armrest, with the wrist hanging over the edge. Raise you hand up as far as possible, using your other hand for assistance if necessary (A). Then lower it as much as possible (B). Repeat with the other hand.

A 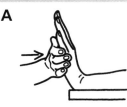 B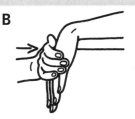

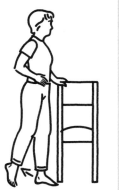

Back kick. Stand facing a table, counter, or the back of a sturdy chair with your hands on it for support. Slowly lift one leg back and up, keeping your knee straight. Hold for a few seconds, then lower. Repeat with the other leg.

Knee bender. Lie on your back on the floor or on a bed with your knees bent. Lift your knee toward your chest. Place your hands on your shin for assistance, and gently bend the knee so that your heel touches your buttock. Hold for a few seconds, then lower and repeat with the other leg.

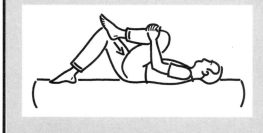

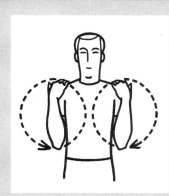

Elbow circles. Stand with your arms at your sides, then slowly bend them up at the elbow until your fingertips touch your shoulders. Then make a large, *gentle* circle with your elbows—bringing them up, out to the sides, down, and then forward again. Breathe in and out with every circle.

Hip stretch. Lie on your back on the floor or on a bed. Bring one knee toward your chest while keeping the other leg straight. Put your hands underneath your thigh for assistance, if necessary. Hold for a few seconds, then lower. Repeat with the other leg.

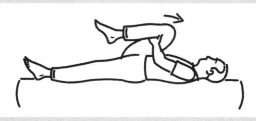

Knee straightener. Sit in a straight-backed chair with one foot resting on another chair or high footstool. Bend your knee slightly, then straighten it by pushing down toward the floor. Repeat with the other leg.

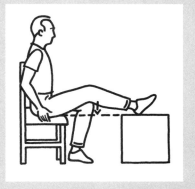

MUSCLE-STRENGTHENING EXERCISES

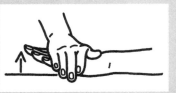

Finger push-up. Place one hand, palm down, on a table and lay the other hand over it, across the fingers. Press the fingers of the bottom hand upward against the top hand and hold. If this is too difficult, lift each finger separately. Switch hand positions and repeat.

Leg lift. Lie on your back on the floor or a bed with your legs straight. Lift one leg up without bending it, keeping the muscles in front of the knee tightened. Hold the leg one to two feet off the floor. Repeat with the other leg. (If this exercise makes your lower back sore, keep the non-exercising knee bent instead of straight.)

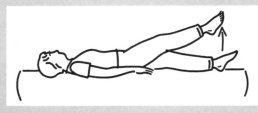

Arm/leg raise. Lie face down on the floor (or a bed) with your arms extended above your head. (Use a small pillow under your stomach and hips to support your back.) Keeping your forehead on the floor, slowly raise your right arm and left leg about four inches off the floor. Repeat the exercise with your left arm and right leg.

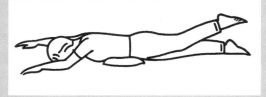

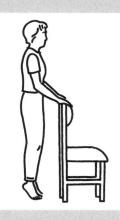

Ankle lift. Stand with your hands on a counter, table, or the back of a sturdy chair for support. Raise yourself up on your toes and hold. Then lower yourself slowly.

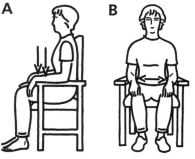

Armrest push. Sit in a chair with armrests, with your wrists hanging over the edge of the armrests. With your palms facing down, press down on the armrests with your forearms and hold (A). Then turn your arms over so that your palms are facing up and repeat. Finally, place your arms at your sides, palms facing down, and press your forearms against the inner sides of the armrests (B).

Sitting leg flex. Sit on the floor with your back supported (against a wall, for example), or on a bed, with your legs extended straight in front of you. In one leg first, and then the other, flex your toes toward your head as you press the back of the knee toward the floor or bed. Hold this position. You should feel the muscle in front of your knee tighten.

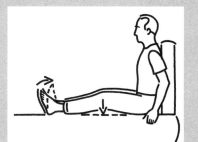

want to exercise, or even move. And while it's important to rest your swollen joints, if you don't keep them moving, they will stiffen and "freeze" until you no longer *can* move them. This can happen gradually, so you don't realize you're losing mobility. But you can preserve your range of motion by moving each joint as far as you can without causing pain. Mild discomfort is okay, however, and if you aren't sure of the difference, ask your doctor or physical therapist to help you recognize it.

It's best to do range-of-motion exercises several times a day: Make them a vital part of your routine. Here are exercises that will help some of your major joints. Do these slowly and carefully.

Start out by doing each exercise three times per session, two to four times a day if possible. Then gradually increase each session to include 10 repetitions of each exercise. Even if the joint is inflamed, you do need to move it (cautiously) so that it won't stiffen up.

Muscle-strengthening. Strong muscles help to prevent pain by supporting your joints and bearing part of the load. Just eight weeks of following a muscle-strengthening program can tone up your muscles and reduce pain significantly. Regular weight lifting builds muscles, of course, but that can be hard on your joints. For many people with arthritis, the answer is called isometrics. These exercises involve pushing or pulling with your muscles but don't actually move or use the joint—so you can get stronger without stressing joints that may be inflamed.

On pages 54-55 is a simple program of exercises that work some of your major muscles without aggravating your joints. Hold each exercise for about six seconds, and do all of them three to four times a day. (But if you have an inflammatory disease such as rheumatoid arthritis, hold off on these exercises during flare-ups.)

Endurance. Gentle aerobic activities such as swimming, walking, and bicycling improve fitness, strengthen joints, and help control your weight without pounding your joints excessively. It's important, however, to warm up before you exercise vigorously and to work gradually into any exercise program. You should get the all-clear from your doctor and perhaps work with a physical therapist to get started. For tips on building your own personal exercise program, look in chapter 10, "An Exercise Program for You."

THE VALUE OF REST

For the average person with osteoarthritis, there's no real need for extra sleep. (Though if it makes you feel better, there's certainly no harm.) However, if you have a severe type of inflammatory arthritis that affects many systems of your body, such as rheumatoid arthritis or lupus that hasn't yet responded to treatment, extra rest can really help. You may need complete bed rest during flare-ups to let the inflammation subside and avoid making it worse. Or, for moderate inflammation, two hours of bed rest daily may be enough. The idea is to continue your rest periods until you feel a significant reduction in your pain for at two weeks. After that, your doctor will probably suggest you cut back on bed rest. Then you can increase your daily activities slowly and cautiously, with appropriate support for arthritic joints that bear your body weight, such as your knees and hips. Here are some other tips.

Relieve pain promptly. Trying to tough it out without pain relief only makes things worse. Either rest your joint, apply heat or cold, or take medication—whichever works for you.

Lie down. You may think you're resting while you're sitting and watching television, but your joints are in a bent position. (Ditto for activities such as driving and gardening.)

Ask your doctor if this may be advisable for you: Relax and stretch the muscles of your hips and knees by stretching out facedown on a firm bed for 15 minutes several times a day. Occasionally you may need to take the pressure off a joint completely to allow it to "rest" and recover.

Use splints and other aids. Using splints, slings, or similar supports also gives joints a time out. Just as a broken bone needs rest and immobility to heal, your inflamed joint may sometimes need the same. Splints, which you can buy ready-made or made to order, support your joint and keep it from moving. This may reduce soreness and keep your muscles from contracting painfully.

But it's important to check first with your doctor about using splints. Even though they can relieve pain, if used incorrectly they can make things worse. Wearing them too often can *weaken* your joint and surrounding muscles. Or, for example, if you sleep with a knee bent over a pillow to ease knee pain (a kind of simple splint), that may ultimately increase your risk of a "frozen joint," or flexion contracture. But depending on your particular condition, your doctor may advise that you wear splints during the night on your hands, wrists, or both. So be sure to heed your doctor's advice and only use such supports as directed.

Your doctor may also advise the use of crutches, a cane, or a walker, possibly temporarily. Although using a walking aid may seem daunting at first, think of it as a handy tool for independence, not a sign of weakness. (You'll find more details on splints and walking aids in chapter 9, "Helping Yourself Live with Arthritis.")

WHAT PHYSICAL THERAPY CAN MEAN TO YOU

Sometimes a physical therapist can seem like a magician, restoring the mobility that you thought was lost long ago. He does this by helping you tune up muscles you may not have known you had, and these muscles can then help support an arthritic joint. He can also help relieve pain that has kept you from using an arm or leg and teach you exercises to strengthen the damaged limb.

Physical therapists can also prescribe items such as braces or wheelchairs, and can help make your home better suit you. A therapist may suggest grab bars in the bathroom or an elevated toilet seat that is easier to sit down on and get up from, for instance. (More information on these and other ideas is coming up in chapter 9.)

All physical therapy programs emphasize exercise. Some exercises are passive, in which the therapist moves your limb for you. In others, you provide some of the motion and the therapist provides the rest. Massage and manipulation are often part of physical therapy. In manipulation, the therapist gently stretches and manipulates your stiff joints to increase their range of motion. Some exercises are resistive, which means you are pushing against a weight—which is sometimes just the therapist's hand.

Other methods of physical therapy also help increase mobility and decrease pain. These include applying heat and cold, such as with heating pads, hot packs, ice bags to reduce swelling, or vapocoolant sprays that numb the skin so a muscle underneath can be gently stretched.

You'll probably enjoy hydrotherapy in a heated pool or whirlpool: Sinking into the warm water can give wonderful relief. And because water helps support your weight, moving in the pool is much easier than when you're high and dry. Gentle exercises in warm water can increase your range of motion and improve your circulation and coordination. Or you may use contrast baths—alternating in cold and hot water—to decrease the swelling of painful hands or feet.

Other treatment methods physical therapists offer include ultrasound and biofeedback. Ultrasound is high-frequency sound waves that penetrate tissue and raise temperature to relieve pain, particularly around tight muscles and tendons. Biofeedback uses electrodes attached to your skin and a device that records and relays electrical signals from your muscle fibers as an audible tone. You use these signals to learn to relax or contract almost any muscle in your body, which in turn helps ease pain.

Some physical therapists may also offer TENS (transcutaneous electrical nerve stimulation), which sends low electrical impulses into painful areas. Although some people believe that TENS eases pain, research studies have actually indicated that this treatment is no more effective than a placebo (a treatment used for comparison that appears the same but actually transmits no current).

WHAT ABOUT "UNCONVENTIONAL" TREATMENTS?

Because some kinds of arthritis can be so overpowering at times, many people understandably strive for some sense of control over the disease—both to obtain peace of mind and to promote healing. Some do this through faith or optimism, some by educating themselves about their disease, some with diet, some with exercise. While all these efforts may indeed be helpful, what may make them seem especially significant is that they are things that you control.

That same positive desire to pitch in and participate in your own arthritis therapy can make you vulnerable to expensive and unproven remedies, however. Especially when things seem to be moving slowly, it's harder to resist the confident claims of many alternative therapies or products that simply don't work. At worst, some may harm you. At best, some may lift your spirits for a while or ease pain momentarily.

If you want to pursue alternative treatments, two concepts are key: You don't want to hurt yourself, and you should

GLUCOSAMINE & CHONDROITIN SULFATE

The author of the best-seller *The Arthritis Cure* recommends a combination of glucosamine and chondroitin sulfate supplements to treat osteoarthritis. These substances, *as they occur naturally in your body*, do help to form and maintain cartilage in your joints. But no one knows yet for sure if the supplements you swallow have the same effect as the products that your body makes.

What concerns most doctors about such claims is that supplements like these are not governed by Food and Drug Administration (FDA) regulations or safeguards as drugs are. That means that health store pitches notwithstanding, you have no guarantees about product purity, because dietary supplements are not tested or regulated. Also, the lack of regulation means you also have no guarantee that the bottle you buy actually contains what it claims on the label.

What's even more important from a medical research perspective, however, is that major, well-designed studies, conducted on large groups of subjects and reported in reputable medical journals, simply have not been done for these substances. Without them, no one is really sure what the safety or side effects of long-term use might be. The medical jury is just not back yet on glucosamine and chondroitin sulfate.

Until reliable research results are in, most doctors recommend putting your money back in your pocket when it comes to these heavily advertised products. If you are still considering using them for your osteoarthritis, however, be sure to discuss it first with your doctor.

never neglect or abandon standard medical care. You also don't want to throw your money away: Alternative treatments are seldom covered by health insurance. While there are reputable alternative practitioners, there are also many who are not—and who are all too happy to relieve you of your money for speculative treatments.

If you choose to visit an alternative therapist, ask for recommendations from friends or doctors, and be sure to ask about credentials and licensing. Bear in mind, however, that most alternative healers can hang out a shingle without extensive training, objective review boards, or any sort of consistent regulation. Unfortunately, it's often a case of "let the buyer beware."

With those warnings in mind, here is a look at alternative practitioners who may have helped some people relieve pain. Unfortunately, there is no scientific evidence that proves these methods are helpful for arthritis. However, some people do feel they have benefited by giving these practitioners a try.

Acupuncturist. In this ancient branch of Chinese medicine, very thin needles are inserted painlessly into the skin to relieve pain or other conditions. Although no one is quite sure how it works, one theory is that acupuncture triggers the release of natural endorphins within the body that act as natural painkillers. Your main concerns are that the acupuncturist is well trained, maintains scrupulous sterilization techniques, and uses disposable needles. (The improper use of needles, whether for acupuncture or tattoos, can transmit hepatitis or even AIDS.) No formal qualification, unfortunately, is required to practice, but there are licensed acupuncturists. Check with the National Commission for the Certification of Acupuncturists (202-232-1401) for help in locating one. Or the American Academy of Medical Acupuncture (800-521-2262) can refer you to a medical doctor who has had at least 200 hours of training in acupuncture. Expect to pay an acupuncturist from $40 to $100 for a first visit and $30 to $70 for each follow-up visit— and more for a medical doctor who also does acupuncture.

Chiropractor. A chiropractor concentrates on adjusting the spine, joints, and muscles, using physical manipulation for therapy. Chiropractic care can be helpful for common low back pain but can be very dangerous for people with ankylosing spondylitis. Manipulation of these people can be fatal. Also, chiropractic should play no role in treating rheumatoid arthritis or lupus, in which the wrong kind of manipulation can cause further pain and damage. Chiropractic treatment may also include massage, application of heat and cold, or TENS—the unproven electrical stimulation method for pain relief that some physical therapists use. A chiropractor should have six years of training at the college level and a state license.

Massage therapist. For sore or overtaxed muscles, massage from a well-trained therapist can feel wonderful. Though it's true that massage can relieve stress and pain in tight muscles, there is no scientific evidence that those good sensations are more than momentary. And they won't make your arthritis disappear. If you enjoy the stress-relieving comfort of massage, there's no harm. But be sure to see only a trained and licensed therapist who also understands the aches and pains of your particular kind of arthritis.

To locate a trained massage therapist, ask your doctor, or call the American Massage Therapy Association, 820 Davis St., Evanston, IL 60201, (708) 864-0123. Prices can range from $30 an hour and up.

Always bear in mind that some types of alternative treatment may not be suited for your particular condition and might even make it worse. So again, before you consider one, be sure to ask your doctor if it will harm you. Whether or not your doctor "believes in" a specific alternative treatment, she can tell you of any possible damaging results. And during any such treatment you do choose to undertake, keep your doctor informed of any changes in your condition.

DON'T WASTE YOUR MONEY ON THESE

So far, no alternative treatment for arthritis has been truly proven to be safe or effective over the long haul. And some have been discredited, including the following.

DMSO (dimethyl sulfoxide). This solvent became a popular folk remedy in the '70s, when people claimed it relieved pain when rubbed on a troublesome joint. You may have known someone who tried it and swore it worked. Maybe it did, in a sense—the brain is pretty powerful, and if you're convinced you're going to feel better, often you do. (Scientists call this the placebo effect, which occurs when people get well even though they have only used a placebo, a "fake" pill containing no medicine.) But controlled studies have found no benefit to DMSO, and it may result in skin irritation or diarrhea. Think about it: This is an *industrial solvent*. Do you really want to rub it on yourself and get it into your system?

Huge doses of vitamins. While some vitamins such as vitamin C are water soluble and any extra you take simply passes through your system and is flushed down the toilet, others are fat soluble and stay in your body. High doses of these can be dangerous. Vitamins D and A in particular can be toxic at high doses. *Never* exceed the recommended daily allowance for these two unless your doctor advises it. (The recommended daily allowance of vitamin D is 400 international units (IU) or 5 micrograms; for vitamin A it's 800 micrograms for women and 1,000 micrograms for men.) You can get vitamin D in enriched milk or from sunlight: It is the one vitamin your body can manufacture itself. About 15 minutes of sun exposure a day is considered adequate. If you want the maximum health benefits of vitamin A, eat foods rich in beta-carotene such as carrots, spinach, sweet potatoes, peaches, and cantaloupe. Beta-carotene converts to vitamin A in the body as it is needed, so you can't overdose on it from food sources. Munch away!

Snake and bee venom injections. Apparently some people get results from bee-sting treatment for diseases such as multiple sclerosis. However, there's no scientific indication that they work for arthritis. (And we don't know that snake bites cure *anything*.) You could have a severe reaction, even if you don't think you're allergic, because the way allergies work you never know when one will flare up. You may not react to your first or 50th sting, but that 51st could trigger a reaction. Play it safe and leave the bees and snakes alone.

"Miracle" drugs. First off, be leery of any product that promises to be a cure-all or miracle drug, especially for arthritis, which can be a complicated ailment. But the major problem for many of these drugs—which may be found in arthritis spas, often along the U.S.-Mexico border—is that they may contain corticosteroids. Steroids do relieve pain, at least for a short time, but they can also cause serious side effects such as ulcers, diabetes, and high blood pressure. So you don't want to take corticosteroids unless absolutely necessary, and then only when you are under the care of a doctor who can monitor you for complications.

CHAPTER 5

What You Eat Can Make a Difference

Is there a special diet for arthritis? There is no quick-fix diet that will magically mend the aches and pains of arthritis. But there's no denying that there is a strong connection between what you eat and how you feel, and that relationship is likely to become more and more apparent the older you get.

What you eat is your body's fuel, and the type of fuel you provide can affect how your arthritis—and, in some cases, your arthritis treatment—affects you.

IS THERE A FOOD CULPRIT?

A simple summary of the direct relationship of food to arthritis goes like this: Diet definitely affects gout, weight loss helps osteoarthritis, and high consumption of fish may ease rheumatoid arthritis. Arthritis related to food allergies is rare, and there's little scientific evidence on any other connection. Here's a closer look at what we know.

Food is clearly a culprit when it comes to gout. Eating large amounts of purines—chemical substances found in alcohol, liver, kidneys, and brains—can trigger attacks of gout. And Reiter's syndrome, another type of arthritis, apparently can develop from eating food or drinking water contaminated by salmonella or other bacteria. (Everyone who encounters these bacteria does not develop arthritis, however. Those who do seem to have a "malfunction" that causes their immune systems to attack their joints rather than the bacteria.)

Food allergies rarely cause arthritis. Some studies have suggested that in a few hypersensitive people, intolerance to foods such as dairy products, alcohol, or preservatives may make arthritis worse or bring on flare-ups. There is little definitive research on this, however, and it's highly individual. But if you think a certain food is triggering your arthritis, it's perfectly sensible to experiment with cutting it out.

Others have suggested that vegetables in the nightshade family, which include tomatoes, potatoes, eggplant, and bell peppers, may aggravate rheumatoid arthritis. No studies prove it, however.

But for most of us, dietary goals need not be so specific. The Arthritis Foundation recommends seven basic diet guidelines:

- Eat a variety of foods.
- Stay at a healthy weight.
- Limit fat and cholesterol.
- Eat lots of vegetables, fruits, and grains.
- Limit sugar.
- Limit salt.
- Limit alcohol.

Generally, a good diet is made up of 15 to 20 percent protein (from lean meats or vegetable sources such as soybeans and other legumes), 25 to 30 percent fat (the healthiest fats are vegetable oils such as olive and canola), and 55 to 60 percent carbohydrates (food such as rice, bread, potatoes, and starchy vegetables like peas and corn). In general, most of us eat too much fat and not enough fruits and vegetables.

HOW TO AVOID OSTEOPOROSIS

Those people with rheumatoid arthritis who take corti‑costeroids, even at low doses, are at risk for osteoporosis, the thinning of our bones that can make them crumble or break. Steroids diminish your body's ability to absorb calcium from the intestines and hamper the manufacture of new bone.

A REASON TO CONSIDER ESTROGEN

Many women are at risk for osteoporosis—some because their bones weren't sturdy enough to start with and some because they get little exercise or don't take in enough calcium or vitamin D, all vital for bone health. When you add to that mix corticosteroids, which are often needed to treat rheumatoid arthritis, lupus, and polymyalgia rheumatica, the risk of osteoporosis soars.

If you need to take corticosteroids and you're post‑menopausal but not taking estrogens, you may want to reconsider. Estrogen is a must for bone building in women. Particularly for small-boned women, many doctors recommend estrogen supplements (called hormone replacement therapy, or HRT, when taken in conjunction with another hormone, progestin) to help protect your bones from thinning.

Supplemental estrogen can also help reduce the risk of osteoarthritis of the hip. Researchers examined the X-rays of 4,000 white women over age 64 and found that those who took estrogen showed 38 percent less osteoarthritis damage. And the protection offered by estrogen apparently increased as time went on. Once a woman stopped estrogen, however, her risk gradually increased again.

It's well accepted that estrogen protects your bones by offsetting osteoporosis. Researchers believe that another way it helps may be by preventing the growths or abnormalities in the bone that osteoporosis can bring, which in turn can damage your cartilage.

Osteoporosis primarily affects the bones of the hip, wrists, and spine. It results in about 1.3 million fractures a year, including spinal fractures in one-third of women older than 65. Preventive measures are particularly important because there are no early warning signs of osteoporosis: The first indications may be a decrease in height or the formation of a dowager's hump as bone in the spine collapses.

Your body borrows calcium daily from your bones for your blood to use. But it also redeposits calcium regularly from the food you eat, so new bone is continually being formed. Around age 40 to 44, the regrowth begins to slow down, and we begin to lose more bone than we manufacture. Add steroids to the mix, and the loss accelerates. To make matters worse, as we get older, it also gets harder for our bodies to absorb calcium—just when we tend to be eating less and in general taking in less calcium in our diets.

Extra vitamin D and calcium, however, can prevent or slow osteoporosis. Most women need 1,500 milligrams of calcium per day, and men need 1,000. The daily requirement for vitamin D is 400 international units (IU), but double that for people older than 50. (Based on blood tests, however, your doctor may recommend a higher dose.)

In a study on rheumatoid arthritis, people on corticosteroids who took supplements of 1,000 milligrams of calcium and 500 IU of vitamin D daily had an *increase* in bone mineral thickness in their lower spines. Those who didn't get the supplements had a 3 percent bone loss each year. (The supplements had no effect on bone thickness in people who didn't take corticosteroids.)

Nutritionists generally recommend trying to get your nutrients through food rather than supplements, however. This is both because you're less likely to overdose on foods and because nutrients may work better when they're in a "package deal"—all wrapped up with other essential nutrients in healthy food. Here are good dietary ways to shore up your stores of calcium and its vital bone-building partner, vitamin D.

Boning Up on Calcium

The best sources of calcium are milk and dairy products. You can choose low-fat or fat-free cheeses, yogurt, or milk. Other good sources are canned salmon and sardines (if you eat the soft bones as well), calcium-fortified orange or grapefruit juice, and broccoli. You can also find smaller amounts of calcium in leafy greens such as kale, collard greens, and turnip greens.

Each serving of cheese, yogurt, or other dairy products equals about 300 milligrams. So if you aim for five servings of calcium-rich foods per day, you'll be getting 1,500 milligrams. If you can't take in that much in food alone, as many people find hard to do, consider a supplement. For best results in preventing osteoporosis, the National Osteoporosis Foundation suggests a supplement of 1,000 to 1,500 milligrams of calcium for people 65 and older; women not taking estrogen need the higher amount.

Other ways to boost your calcium intake: Add nonfat dry milk to hot cereals, stews, casseroles, meat loaf, or mashed potatoes; use ricotta cheese or cottage cheese as a sandwich filling or spread on toast; replace beef or chicken in stir-fry recipes with tofu, or soybean curd; add tofu, or soybean curd, to salads; have low-fat milkshakes instead of soft drinks.

And while you're upping your intake, you'll also want to slow your calcium "out-take," or loss, in the following ways.

Limit coffee. One study showed that middle-aged women who drank more than six cups of coffee a day had three times the risk of hip fracture than those who drank less than a cup and a half a day. Caffeine may harm your bones directly, or indirectly by making you urinate more often, which increases the amount of calcium you lose in your urine. It's wise to cut your coffee intake or consider making the switch to decaf.

Cut back on alcohol. Alcohol can interfere with your ability to absorb and use calcium. Because women's ovaries are sensitive to alcohol, it can alter the hormonal balance necessary for strong bones. And alcohol's diuretic qualities may also promote more calcium loss through the urine.

Watch your soda intake. The amount of phosphorus in your diet may affect how much calcium you can obtain from your food. Some studies suggest that large amounts of sodas, which contain phosphoric acid, can limit the calcium you'll have available. One survey found that women who drank carbonated drinks had more than twice as many broken bones as those who didn't drink soda. It won't hurt to limit your soda intake to one can a day or less.

Don't Forget the Sunshine Vitamin

Vitamin D is important in building bones and keeping them strong. Without enough vitamin D, bone and the cartilage that covers it may not recover fully after an injury or blow. Vitamin D is found in green leafy vegetables such as kale and collard greens and in egg yolks and enriched milk.

Your body can also manufacture vitamin D from exposure to sunlight. This is tricky, as you don't want to risk sunburn or excessive sun exposure, but researchers estimate that 10 to 15 minutes of sunlight can provide enough sun to help your bones. (It's best to spend this time outdoors in early morning or late afternoon, thus avoiding the hours when the sun's damaging rays are strongest.) You can also get the recommended daily allowance of 400 IU from two glasses of enriched milk.

FATTY ACIDS AND YOU

Neither "fatty" nor "acid" is a word we commonly associate with something good, but some fatty acids play important roles in our health. In your body, they change to substances called prostaglandins, which are crucial in telling different kinds of cells (such as intestinal, kidney, and lung cells) how to function.

Cold-water fish such as salmon, mackerel, and herring are high in omega-3 fatty acids, which convert in your body to prostaglandins that apparently can help prevent heart disease and reduce the harmful blood fats called triglycerides. There's some evidence that the prostaglandins from omega-3s also slow rheumatoid arthritis. In an Australian study, 23 people who took fish oil daily for three months found that their joints were less sore and they could grip things more tightly than they could before the study. Experts recommend eating cold-water fish at least twice a week, and more often if possible. These include mackerel, tuna, salmon, sardines, herring, cod, and bluefish.

THE ARTHRITIS DIET

If there were a magic diet that was guaranteed to ease your arthritis pain, would you follow it?

You bet you would.

For many arthritis sufferers, losing weight—even if you're only mildly overweight—can help ease the pain and protect your joints. Think about it: The more pressure and weight on your joints, the more they hurt. Even 10 extra pounds stresses a joint that much more. This is more significant for people with osteoarthritis; many people with rheumatoid arthritis, in fact, lose their appetites, sometimes because of their medication. Nevertheless, eating a well-balanced diet *is* crucial for people with rheumatoid arthritis.

ALCOHOL AND YOU

If you are taking aspirin or other nonsteroidal anti-inflammatory drugs (NSAIDs) or corticosteroids, stomach problems such as ulcers are more likely if you also drink alcohol. Too much acetaminophen (such as Tylenol) along with alcohol can damage the liver seriously, and the medication methotrexate plus alcohol can also cause liver damage. Also, alcohol can make agonizing gout attacks happen more frequently, because it can increase the level of uric acid in your blood. Always ask your doctor how much, if any, drinking is safe for you.

Before you try to limit your foods or go on a diet, talk to your doctor. He may refer you to a nutritionist, who can help guide you to an easy way to weight loss. Nutritionists will tell you that "diets" don't work, and if you've tried them you'll likely agree. The diets touted in many magazines or on television may result in quick weight loss—sometimes too quick to be healthy—but they are generally so extreme that you can't stay on them for long. And when you return to your "regular eating," the pounds leap back on.

You don't need to go on a deprivation diet; you need to *permanently* change to a healthy, delicious, balanced way of eating. Quite likely, you'll also be making changes in how you shop and cook (and you'll build exercise into your daily life, if you haven't already). It sounds like a big undertaking—and it does require commitment—but a nutritionist can ease the way. You've got great motivation, don't forget—whittling down the discomforts of arthritis along with your waistline. And don't worry, a good nutritionist will find room in your diet for your favorite foods. If you've got to have chocolate, you'll be able to work it in (just probably not every day and not in large amounts!).

Once you start your new routine, don't be surprised if it takes three weeks or so before you begin to see results. Our bodies tend to be stubborn, and they instinctively *like* to hold on to the status quo—the weight they've got. Just hang in there! You'll eventually begin to lose. And slow weight loss (one to two pounds per week) is safest: If you lose *more* than two pounds a week, begin to eat a little more.

Here's a simple, basic meal plan you can adjust for your needs.

Breakfast. One piece or serving of fresh fruit; one slice of bread or bowl of cereal; one protein such as an egg or a cup of yogurt.

Lunch. A fresh salad with vegetables such as mushrooms, carrots, tomatoes, radishes, and celery and low-fat dressing; a protein such as a four-ounce serving of fish, chicken, turkey, tofu, or beans; one bread serving; a piece of fresh fruit.

Afternoon snack. One fruit or raw vegetable; one bread; a glass of low-fat milk or a cup of low-fat yogurt.

Dinner. A four-ounce serving of protein such as fish, tofu, chicken, beans, turkey, beef; one carbohydrate such as a baked potato, rice, bread, or pasta; one cup of steamed vegetables (not starchy ones such as peas or corn); a fresh salad with low-fat dressing.

Evening snack. One fruit with one square of graham cracker, one low-fat cookie, or a half cup of sorbet or low-fat frozen yogurt.

And don't forget that the real dessert for your body is *exercise.* While you're eating healthy meals, to start burning fat, exercise for at least 20 minutes three to four times a week, walking, swimming, or whatever, as your arthritis allows. If you can exercise longer, however, you'll do much better: Your body burns mostly carbohydrates during that first 20 minutes and doesn't begin to use up stored fat until *after* 20 minutes.

TEN TIPS TO MAKE EATING WELL EASY

Remember this simple rule: It takes three weeks to make something a habit, and some people report that it takes at least six weeks to adjust to low-fat and lower-calorie eating. So if you find yourself wavering, wait it out—it's worth it. Here are some tips to help.

Allow yourself treats. Eat whatever you crave, but just don't eat much of it. If you think you will die if you don't have some chocolate, walk or bike to the store and buy a tiny chocolate bar and eat it. Otherwise you can eat celery until you turn into a giant stalk, but you still won't be happy.

Pack your lunch. If you work a 9-to-5 job, it's tough to get a fast, healthy lunch during your brief lunch hour. You're better off packing your own. A sandwich with low-fat meat, water-packed tuna, or tofu spread, plus fruit and carrot sticks will fill you up and keep you going all afternoon. You can get a lunch container with ice packs if you don't want to trust your food to the company fridge.

Try something new. Experiment with low-cal substitutes for your favorite foods. Maybe you can put mushrooms in tomato sauce instead of meatballs and sausage. Eat sherbet instead of ice cream. Savor a graham cracker instead of a cookie (you loved them when you were little).

Read labels. You'll think twice about devouring fast-food fries when you read the chart on the wall and discover that an order has 25 grams of fat—a huge chunk of your daily allotment. And when you see the calorie count of those low-fat cookies (remember, *low-fat* doesn't mean *low-calorie*), you may put them back on the shelf. Also, foods such as cereal vary greatly in calorie and fat content. If you buy a cereal loaded with nuts and dried fruit, one serving is only a tiny heap. Instead, purchase a basic cereal such as shredded wheat or bran flakes and flavor it with a bit of the "fancy" kind.

Make special orders. You can enjoy eating out and care for yourself at the same time. Read the menu carefully and ask things like, "Does this chicken come without skin?" and "Can you serve those vegetables without butter?" and say "Dressing on the side, please."

Use small plates and small bowls. This is purely psychological, but it works. You feel better starting out with a full plate rather than a large one with the food rattling around on it. Likewise, when you have frozen desserts such as sherbet, use a tiny bowl.

Get a decent, digital scale. The other kind encourages too much fudging (Hey, if you lean way to the left, you've lost five pounds!). Weigh yourself at regular intervals and record your weight. This keeps you honest and helps you stay aware of your goal.

Never skip meals—especially breakfast! When you wake up, your body is in "low gear" and burning few calories. If you don't eat, your body thinks you're starving and stays at that low-calorie-burning rate. Eating actually "revs up" your engine and starts your metabolism burning calories faster.

Substitute when you cook. Instead of frying, broil foods or sauté them in broth. Use applesauce instead of Crisco, butter, or margarine and egg substitutes or egg whites instead of whole eggs. Also, in most recipes you can cut the sugar by at least one-third. Forget about using mixes for cakes or muffins, because you can't adjust the recipe. But for most unyeasted baked goods, it's surprisingly easy to do things the old-fashioned way: Mix flour and a few other ingredients, and you're done!

Change how you shop. Avoid or limit high-fat foods such as sunflower seeds, avocados, nuts, crackers, pizza, creamy soups or casseroles, cheese and cream cheese, sour cream, butter or margarine, sausage, and pepperoni. Good choices include low-fat or nonfat salad dressing, low-fat lunch meats, nonfat milk, nonfat or low-fat cheese, egg substitute, water-packed tuna, tofu, and canned or dried legumes such as pinto beans, kidney beans, and split peas.

INTERACTIONS WITH YOUR MEDICATIONS

Your doctor has undoubtedly warned you about the hazards of side effects from your medications. However, an often overlooked side effect is the effect of medication on your *nutrient* status.

Here are some common problems that can result and the simple solutions.

Problem: Some antacids can have high levels of sodium, calcium, and magnesium. Too much calcium may cause kidney stones and can interfere with your body's use of other important minerals such as iron and zinc. It can also cause a dangerous condition called hypercalcemia, which can damage kidney function. Excess magnesium can trigger diarrhea.

Solution: Talk it over with your doctor. Based on your medical history, she will know whether you need to modify your intake of antacids or perhaps have your blood tested to see if they are causing problems.

Problem: Antacids with aluminum or magnesium hydroxide may lower your level of phosphorus, which you need to use calcium.

Solution: Choose another antacid or include lean meat and poultry in your diet for an adequate phosphorus supply.

Problem: Corticosteroid medicines may cause you to lose potassium, absorb less vitamin D, and retain sodium. Potassium and vitamin D are both crucial nutrients.

Solution: Good sources of potassium include prune juice, carrot juice, orange juice, baked potatoes, avocados, bananas, clams, nonfat yogurt, and many raw fruits and vegetables.

You can get vitamin D in enriched milk, tuna, and salmon and through exposure to sunlight. Decrease your salt intake to help compensate for the retained sodium.

Problem: Colchicine, a gout medication, can affect how vitamin B_{12} is absorbed.

Solution: You can enjoy a boost of vitamin B_{12} in tuna, oysters, and beef (lean, of course).

Problem: Methotrexate, a common treatment for rheumatoid arthritis, may interfere with your body's use of folic acid, an important nutrient. This, in turn, can contribute to methotrexate toxicity, which can damage your liver.

Solution: Your doctor will routinely prescribe folic acid supplements if you're on methotrexate, but you can also find folic acid in wheat germ, liver, oranges, orange juice, eggs, milk, navy and lima beans, spinach, asparagus, and broccoli.

Problem: Grapefruit juice has been found to have a major effect on absorption of several medicines, including cyclosporin for rheumatoid arthritis.

Solution: Ask your doctor whether any of your medications are affected by grapefruit juice. If the answer is yes, switch to orange juice. Better yet, get your nutrients from whole fruit, which is nutritionally far superior to juices.

CHAPTER 6

Medications to Fight Arthritis

You may feel reluctant about medication; lots of us do. But if you have arthritis, the right medication can feel like a miracle.

With osteoarthritis, medication can relieve pain and swelling, allowing you to continue using your joints and keep them flexible and mobile. The most common and safest medication for osteoarthritis is over-the-counter acetaminophen (one brand is Tylenol), and some people find additional relief with a rub-on medication or cream such as Zostrix. If these two don't do the job, your doctor may recommend drugs such as aspirin, ibuprofen (such as Advil or Nuprin), or naproxen (Aleve). Occasionally, injected corticosteroids may be needed to relieve the pain and inflammation. Later in this chapter, we'll discuss all these medicines in more detail.

Rheumatoid arthritis, a far more virulent disease, must be treated more aggressively to minimize the potential damage to your joints. Medications used for treatment include nonsteroidal anti-inflammatory drugs (NSAIDs), corticosteroids, slow-acting anti-rheumatic drugs (SAARDs), and low-dose antidepressants (to relieve pain and improve the quality of your sleep).

QUESTIONS TO ASK YOUR DOCTOR ABOUT NEW MEDICATION

Your medicine will help you most if you're sure how to use it properly. To get the complete picture, ask your doctor:

- ◆ What time of day should I take this medication?
- ◆ Should I take it with meals?
- ◆ What should I do if I forget to take it one day?
- ◆ Will any food or drink interfere with how the medication works?
- ◆ What side effects might I experience?
- ◆ What should I do if side effects do occur?
- ◆ Do any of my current medications, prescription or nonprescription, interfere with this medicine?
- ◆ How long will I be taking this drug?
- ◆ Can I take over-the-counter remedies such as Tums or Advil with this medication?
- ◆ Is there a generic equivalent I could use?

OVER-THE-COUNTER MEDICATION MAY BE THE ANSWER

For many years doctors routinely prescribed NSAIDs (pronounced "en-seds") for osteoarthritis. But these drugs can have uncomfortable side effects, and people with osteoarthritis pain don't always need an anti-inflammatory. Unlike the pain of rheumatoid arthritis and similar conditions, where the underlying problem is inflammation, the pain of osteoarthritis can be caused by muscles in spasm or bone problems, for example. While anti-inflammatories may relieve the pain, they also have a greater chance of causing ulcers and other complications. One study found that for many people with osteoarthritis, over-the-counter pain relievers such as acetaminophen or low-dose ibuprofen worked just as well as more potent—and more expensive—

prescription anti-inflammatories. (You will find a more detailed look at NSAIDs, how they work, and how best to use them, beginning on page 84.)

For many people with osteoarthritis, acetaminophen, which you probably know best as Tylenol, is safe and is the only drug you need. Acetaminophen relieves pain but is not an anti-inflammatory. Therefore, it lacks the side effects such as stomach upset and ulcers that sometimes go hand in hand with anti-inflammatory action.

But acetaminophen *can* cause problems for some people. Taking more than the recommended amounts can cause kidney disease: One study showed that taking more than one acetaminophen pill a day or more than 1,000 pills during your life doubles your chance of kidney failure. And acetaminophen combined with alcohol can damage your liver, so you should never take it when you're drinking. While you're taking acetaminophen, be sure your doctor monitors you for side effects.

If acetaminophen isn't effective, your doctor may advise aspirin or ibuprofen (Advil or Motrin) instead. In low doses, these act primarily as pain relievers; in higher or prescription doses, they are anti-inflammatories. Even at low doses they may cause stomach upset or ulcers, however, so use them cautiously.

TINGLY SALVES AND SUCH

Products such as Ben-Gay or Absorbine Jr. may ease some of the pain of osteoarthritis and related problems such as tendinitis (but won't help with rheumatoid arthritis). Here's what they can do and how to use them.

Counterirritants. The warm or cool feeling you get from the product can trick your mind into forgetting about the pain for a bit. These products contain camphor, menthol, or turpentine oil. You can apply them three or four times a day, but if you're reaching for the tube more than a few times a week, your doctor may need to modify your treatment program so that you aren't in such pain.

These topical treatments may also contain salicylates (a group of drugs that includes aspirin). One study found that salicylates from creams applied daily were absorbed into the skin. If you are sensitive to salicylates or are taking medication such as warfarin that could interact with salicylates, use these salves with caution. Symptoms of a salicylate overdose include blurred vision, shortness of breath, and ringing in the ears. If you experience any of these, call your doctor.

Capsaicin products. Products containing capsaicin relieve pain directly. They apparently interfere with the neurotransmitters that carry pain "messages" from your nerves to your brain. Capsaicin, the same ingredient that makes hot peppers hot, is available over the counter in an ointment called Zostrix. If you use it, stay with it. It must be applied three or four times a day and will start to take effect after two to six weeks. You should not, of course, use any of these peppery products on skin that has an open cut or apply them near your eyes, nose, or mouth.

The Next Step for OA

For a few people with osteoarthritis, the milder methods of pain relief, such as exercise, diet, salves, acetaminophen, or low-dose aspirin or ibuprofen, simply aren't enough. They may need a stronger or different drug or one that will help relieve inflammation. Here are other possible treatments.

NSAIDs. These drugs, which include high-dose ibuprofen and aspirin, work by lowering the amount of a substance called prostaglandin that causes inflammation, joint pain, and stiffness. The downside is that because prostaglandins help protect your stomach, when their levels

AT HOME WITH OSTEOARTHRITIS

If you have rheumatoid arthritis or another inflammatory disease, your medication regimen will be precisely detailed by your doctor. With osteoarthritis, however, things aren't always so clear. Say you're at home and your arthritic knee begins to hurt. What do you do?

1. The first step is simple: Stop what you're doing, and take your weight off the knee.

2. Apply ice to relieve the pain. (Hot packs or a hot bath work better for some people, so try these if ice doesn't do the job.)

3. If it still hurts, you may want to try a rub-on product such as Zostrix to relieve the pain.

4. Still hurting? If you need medication, it's probably best to try acetaminophen (Tylenol) first, as it has the least chance of causing side effects.

5. It's the next day, and you're still in pain? It's time to try aspirin or ibuprofen (Advil or Aleve).

6. No relief yet? Your doctor may prescribe a nonsteroidal anti-inflammatory drug (NSAID) or advise taking ibuprofen in higher doses. Because of potential side effects, however, you don't want to use NSAIDs casually, whether they are prescription or nonprescription.

7. If pain continues or worsens, your doctor may discuss the possibility of surgery. (You'll find details in chapter 8.)

8. Once you've gotten better, your final step is to build a regular stretching, muscle-strengthening, and exercise program into your daily life to help prevent further problems. You'll feel better for it! (Chapter 10 gives tips on starting your exercise program.)

drop, your stomach acid is more likely to damage your stomach lining. Fortunately, as inflammation isn't a major problem with osteoarthritis, you won't need the NSAIDs with the strongest inflammation-fighting effect (which are also those with the strongest side effects). But stomach problems can still occur.

The good news? New NSAIDs that inhibit inflammation without harming the stomach are being developed. In the meantime, here's how to help protect yourself.

- Stop smoking and limit alcohol, especially on an empty stomach.
- Take pills with a large glass of water and something to eat.
- If you use aspirin, choose the enteric-coated variety. The coating lets the pill pass through your stomach before dissolving in the less fragile small intestine.
- Don't miss your prescribed dosage and never double up if you miss a dose.

And you don't want to overuse NSAIDs—prescription or nonprescription—or take them lightly. Large doses of NSAIDs can contribute to high blood pressure and kidney damage, especially in people with heart failure or kidney problems or who take diuretics. Though researchers don't agree, it is also possible that NSAIDs speed cartilage breakdown or slow the formation of new cartilage. And they may relieve your pain so well that you're tempted to work your joints more than you should. (Pain, while it's no fun, does remind you that something is wrong and that you need to take it easy.) For all these reasons, your doctor should monitor your use of any NSAID.

Corticosteroid injections. For severe flare-ups of osteoarthritis or for a joint so badly damaged that you may need a joint replacement, your doctor may inject adrenal corticosteroids into your joint. This can relieve your pain for as long as several months, an important benefit, because this allows you to start physical therapy to strengthen your joint. Having these injections more than several times a year, however, increases the risk of damage to cartilage. Corticosteroids relieve pain by reducing inflammation, so if the pain returns in a few weeks, you can probably rule out inflammation as the primary problem.

WHEN TO SEEK MEDICAL HELP

Sometimes you may develop an allergy to medication. If you faint or develop rapid breathing, or wheezing, or a rapid heartbeat, have someone whisk you to the emergency room or call 911.

A more common problem than allergy with arthritis medication is an ulcer, or a small hole in the stomach lining that may bleed. If you vomit or spit up blood or have a very dark or black stool (which could also be from bleeding), you should call your doctor immediately. Ulcers can cause stomach pain, but it's also possible to develop bleeding from an ulcer without any pain. That may be because, ironically, the NSAID that produced the problem eases pain and so also prevents you from feeling it. The early warning signs of ulcers that you can easily detect, however, include:

- Stomach pain that goes away if you take antacids or eat
- Stomach cramps
- Severe heartburn
- Nausea or vomiting

NSAIDs may sometimes cause you to retain fluid as well. These symptoms include sudden weight gain; swollen ankles, feet, or legs; shortness of breath; and unexplained fatigue. If you have any of these problems, you should stop taking your NSAID and call your doctor right away.

TREATING INFLAMMATORY DISEASES

When it comes to rheumatoid arthritis and other inflammatory conditions, treatment is a different ball game. In rheumatoid arthritis, your well-meaning (but misguided) white blood cells rush to the joint to "protect" it against the supposed invader or injury. In the process, they release chemicals that inflame the synovium, or joint-lining membrane, which makes the joint red, swollen, and painful. The membrane thickens, and a mass can grow on the cartilage. When this happens, the mass in turn produces substances that can erode the cartilage and damage bones, tendons, and ligaments.

If you like to avoid medication at all costs, now is the time to rethink your position. The sobering truth is that untreated rheumatoid arthritis can be a crippling disease and, at its worst, could give you about the same life expectancy as people with leukemia or advanced heart disease. And without medication, you may not live as long or as comfortably as most. What's crucial to understand, however, is that multiple studies indicate that early, aggressive drug therapy makes a major difference. Without it, half of the people with rheumatoid arthritis are unable to get around on their own after six years, and 9 out of 10 reach this state after two decades. But early treatment can greatly change the outcome.

The main goals of treatment are to:

◆ Relieve pain
◆ Reduce inflammation
◆ Maintain function
◆ Prevent deformities

Because 90 percent of the joint damage occurs in the first few years of rheumatoid arthritis, it's vital not to delay treatment. Again, many doctors believe that beginning treatment right away, and aggressively, can significantly reduce the damage to your joints.

If you are fortunate, NSAIDs such as aspirin at an anti-inflammatory dosage may be all you need. If you have more aggressive rheumatoid arthritis, however, you may need the stronger agents called slow-acting antirheumatic drugs (SAARDs). These include disease-modifying antirheumatic drugs (DMARDs), plus immunosuppressive medications (which suppress immune system cells). SAARDs are aimed at controlling inflammation, and though they take awhile longer to work, in the end they are more powerful than NSAIDs.

DMARDS include oral or injected gold, hydroxychloroquine, sulfasalazine, and penicillamine. The immunosuppressive drugs include methotrexate, azathioprine, cyclosporin, cyclophosphamide, and corticosteroids.

Your doctor may also recommend antidepressants such as amitriptyline (Elavil) and nortriptyline (Pamelor) for you. Taken in smaller doses than when prescribed for depression, antidepressants block pain messengers in the brain and help restore your normal sleep patterns.

We'll discuss all these drugs, one by one, starting with the simplest—aspirin.

ASPIRIN CAN BE YOUR FRIEND

Aspirin is the cheapest of the drugs used to treat rheumatoid arthritis and may be the first drug your doctor will suggest. But because different people use aspirin in their bodies at different rates, the dosage you need may be quite different from your neighbor's or even from what the label suggests. Your doctor will probably gradually increase your dosage until you improve significantly or begin to have side effects and then adjust it downward.

One of the first side effects that may appear is ringing in the ears, also called tinnitus. This will go away when your doctor decreases the dosage. Aspirin also can interfere with the platelets in your blood, which are involved in clotting, so you may find that you bruise more easily. Other side effects can include nausea and vomiting or ulcers.

Years ago, when aspirin appeared on your shopping list, it was easy. You grabbed one giant bottle, maybe the only kind available, which may have cost less than a dollar. Today you have a lot more choices, which can be pretty confusing. While aspirin is aspirin—and generic is just fine—manufacturers do prepare it in different ways, which can affect how effective or useful it will be.

You'll probably do better if you take aspirin with meals. Because aspirin is a salicylate, it can contribute to stomach ulcers. One good alternative, particularly if you need to take aspirin frequently, is to choose enteric-coated tablets, which dissolve in the small intestine rather than the stomach. Another may be to try a related drug called salsalate, which is less likely to irritate your stomach than aspirin (but may irritate your wallet some, as it does cost more). Occasionally, someone who is allergic to aspirin may have trouble with salsalate as well, so be sure to check with your doctor.

REDUCING THE SIDE EFFECTS OF NSAIDS

The NSAIDs prescribed for inflammatory diseases are likely to be the stronger ones, and they can cause serious side effects in some people, particularly the elderly. As we mentioned earlier, the most common problems are stomach irritation and ulcers, or sores on your stomach lining that may bleed. Regular use of NSAIDs can also cause other gastrointestinal troubles such as indigestion, stomach pain, and diarrhea. Fortunately, more serious consequences, such as colitis, are much less common. Very, very rarely, kidney or liver failure is possible.

The differences between various NSAIDs are hotly debated. Ibuprofen in low doses is probably the safest. Reports on the differences between the other types, and there are many, vary from research study to study. All NSAIDs, however, can potentially cause some side effects. Because the NSAID picture can be confusing, as you work with your doctor, hang in there. Although you may need to try more than one kind, you'll eventually find the one that works best for you.

DRUGS THAT MAY
INTERACT WITH NSAIDS

You should tell your doctor about any medication you are taking, even if it is over-the-counter (nonprescription). These drugs may cause problems if you take NSAIDs:

- ACE inhibitors (Lotensin, Capoten, Vasotec)
- Anticoagulants (Coumadin)
- Azathioprine (Imuran)
- Beta-blockers (Tenormin, Lopressor, Inderal)
- Corticosteroids (prednisone)
- Diabetes drugs taken by mouth (Dymelor, Diabinese, Glucotrol)
- Digoxin (Lanoxicaps, Lanoxin)
- Diuretics (Lasix, Esidrix, HydroDIURIL, Lozol)
- Lithium (Eskalith, Lithobid)
- Metoclopramide (Octamide, Reglan)
- Penicillamine (Cuprimine, Depen)
- Phenytoin sodium (Dilantin)
- Probenecid (Benemid)

Avoiding overuse. Realize that if you should take an over-the-counter medication such as aspirin or ibuprofen in addition to your prescribed NSAID, you would be essentially increasing your NSAID dosage—and therefore increasing your risk of side effects. It's unwise to be taking two NSAIDs at once. So, if you need pain relief in addition to your prescribed medication, acetaminophen is the safer choice. (And, of course, be sure to clear any over-the-counter medication with your doctor.)

Staying in touch with your doctor. Report any signs of gastrointestinal problems to your doctor right away. These include vomiting blood or having a black, tarry stool. Signs of an ulcer include severe heartburn or stomach cramps, nausea or vomiting, and stomach pains that disappear if you take antacids.

Considering alternative drugs. Fortunately, if you have unavoidable risk factors for ulcers but you nonetheless need NSAIDs, there are additional medications that can reduce your chances of ulcer problems. One such drug is misoprostol (Cytotec). In a six-month study of people with rheumatoid arthritis, the misoprostol helped reduce gastrointestinal side effects caused by taking NSAIDs. Those most vulnerable are men over 65 who have had peptic ulcers, use antacids, or have heart disease. Misoprostol reduced gastrointestinal problems in all these categories. Ironically, misoprostol itself can sometimes cause diarrhea, nausea, and stomach pain. One study found, however, that taking the 200-microgram dosage two to three times a day rather than four times reduced those side effects and was still effective. Another ulcer-blocking drug is famotidine (Pepcid), which is prescribed in doses of 40 milligrams to prevent ulcers (twice the usual dose of 20 milligrams).

The Scoop on the SAARDs

SAARDs are very effective medicines that may be just what the doctor ordered for your individual arthritis situation. Some do carry more risk of side effects, however. Because of the possible toxicity of some of these drugs, you'll get the best results if you take them exactly as directed, keep notes on how you're feeling, and report your progress and any problems to your doctor.

Methotrexate. This medication is the "star" of inflammation-fighting drugs because of its rapid action and its relative lack of side effects. In the usual doses it only mildly suppresses the immune system and reduces inflammation. Improvement can appear within a month but may take longer. Methotrexate is taken by mouth once a week. Side effects include stomach irritation and inflammation of the lining in your mouth. In a few people, it can cause lung inflammation, bone marrow problems, and serious liver effects. To reduce the risk of liver damage, it's best to drink no alcohol while on methotrexate. Blood tests will be recommended every four to eight weeks to monitor the health of your liver. And because, like many arthritis medications, methotrexate may potentially cause birth defects, it should be avoided during pregnancy. Very rarely, your doctor might suggest a liver biopsy to check for damage.

A simple dietary strategy can help you: low doses of folic acid, a B vitamin that's plentiful in fresh spinach, wheat germ, and other foods. In many studies, daily folic acid reduces side effects from methotrexate. In fact, doctors routinely prescribe a folic acid supplement to make sure you'll be getting enough. Many doctors think methotrexate is the best choice for rheumatoid arthritis when NSAIDs aren't effective.

Antimalarials. Hydroxychloroquine sulfate (Plaquenil) is the most common SAARD. Around a third of people with rheumatoid arthritis will benefit after using it for three to six months on a dose of 200 to 400 milligrams daily. This SAARD has few side effects; the most serious possible risk, though rare, is damage to the retina of your eye. However, eye damage is uncommon at the usual doses, and because your doctor will recommend that you step up your eye exam schedule to twice a year, it can likely be avoided. Gastrointestinal side effects are also possible.

Corticosteroids. These include cortisone and prednisone and are prescribed for rheumatoid arthritis as well as other inflammatory diseases such as lupus. They rapidly reduce inflammation and suppress the immune system that's mistakenly causing your body to "attack" itself. If you have such severe rheumatoid arthritis that you can't get up and go, or you're waiting for other drugs such as DMARDs to take effect, nothing is more effective at putting you back in motion. Corticosteroids are also advisable in cases of severe internal inflammation, such as vasculitis. The inflammation may return if you stop taking them, however.

Long-term steroid use can cause side effects, most commonly weight gain. That's because they can give you an incredible appetite for sweets. To prevent the extra pounds, therefore, it's crucial to weigh yourself daily, avoid excess sugar, and exercise all you safely can.

Along with weight gain, some people on corticosteroids develop a group of symptoms including a round, red face, a rise in blood pressure, and frequent bruising. Other side effects can include stomach ulcers, diabetes, poor wound healing, acne, muscle weakening, and cataracts. There's also an increased risk of osteoporosis, so taking measures to prevent bone loss is very important. (See "How to Avoid

Osteoporosis," page 69.) And if you take these drugs for a long time, your body will stop making its own naturally occurring corticosteroids that battle infection, so your doctor will monitor you for any infection problems. Finally, if you're on long-term corticosteroids, you should wear a medical alert bracelet in case of an accident, as emergency doctors sometimes need to give replacement steroids.

Sulfasalazine. A new, delayed-release medication for rheumatoid arthritis is sulfasalazine, a combination of a sulfa drug and a salicylate. It suppresses the haywire immune system and helps fight the inflammation that's already present. Usually your doctor will prescribe two grams daily, and you'll notice the effect of sulfasalazine in about four weeks. Occasional side effects can include rash, headache, nausea, vomiting, loss of appetite, stomach problems, and low sperm count. Sulfasalazine's results are considered comparable to those of gold salts and penicillamine. If you take sulfasalazine, your doctor will want you to have frequent complete blood counts.

Gold salts. If NSAIDs don't help and you can't take methotrexate, your doctor may try gold salts, which can delay or prevent bone erosion. (They help about 6 people out of 10.) You won't see the benefits for three to six months, however, so treatment requires patience. You take the gold either by weekly injections into your muscles or by pills twice a day. About a third of those who use gold experience side effects. These can include a rash, inflammation of the mouth, protein in the urine (which may signal kidney problems), and a decrease in both red and white blood cells. Less commonly, gold may also lower platelets in the blood. Gold can also cause diarrhea, plus dizziness and nausea from the injections. Discuss any problems you're having with your doctor, who will also do regular blood tests to monitor side effects.

Minocycline. This mildly effective agent is used only for mild cases of rheumatoid arthritis. No one is sure just how it works, but it does fight inflammation and apparently inhibits the enzymes that destroy cartilage. The only significant side effect of minocycline is that about 1 in 10 people may feel dizzy after taking it.

Penicillamine. Studies in England have shown that penicillamine helps people with severe rheumatoid arthritis when nothing else does. About half may experience side effects, which can include fever, rash, mouth ulcers, loss of taste, protein in the urine, and low levels of white blood cells and platelets, which your doctor will monitor with blood tests. You should never use penicillamine if you are pregnant, as it can cause birth defects.

Azathioprine (Imuran). This medication works by suppressing the immune reaction that causes inflammation and is often used to prevent the body's rejection of heart or kidney transplants. It's not known exactly how it works in rheumatoid arthritis, however. Because azathioprine's effect on your immunity can make you more vulnerable to infection, it's generally used when alternatives such as antimalarials and gold do not work. Side effects can include loss of appetite, nausea, and sometimes vomiting, and because it can cause birth defects, it must be avoided during pregnancy. Azathioprine takes several months to be effective.

Cyclosporin (CyA). This drug suppresses the immune system and relieves symptoms of inflammation. It can cause kidney damage, so you can take only low doses, and your doctor must monitor you closely. One study showed that cyclosporin controlled damage to joints better than other treatments: After a year, people treated with CyA had less bone erosion than those who were treated with other DMARDs. Only about 11 percent of the CyA group showed new bone erosion at the end of the year, while the bones of more than half of the people on other medications had eroded.

Cyclophosphamide (Cytoxan). In experimental studies, Cytoxan, a drug used to fight cancer, helped rheumatoid arthritis when nothing else did. Apparently it binds to DNA and RNA and inhibits cell reproduction—and that includes the reproduction of haywire immune system cells. Bladder inflammation is a side effect, however, so if you take Cytoxan, be sure to drink lots of water. This drug can damage developing babies, so pregnant women should not take it. Also, Cytoxan use can increase the risk of developing cancer later in life.

SOME OF THE MOST COMMON NSAIDS

Overall, NSAIDs do not differ greatly in effectiveness or toxicity (the potential for side effects). In most cases the biggest difference between types of NSAIDs is in their cost or their convenience—some offer dosage schedules of once or twice a day versus four times, for example.

Most NSAIDs are equally effective in treating arthritis, with the exception of Indocin, which is more effective for akylosing spondylitis and possibly for osteoarthritis of the hip.

The most common side effects of NSAIDs, gastrointestinal irritation (nausea, vomiting) and ulcers, are least likely to occur with ibuprofen. All the rest cause roughly similar levels of side effects, with a few exceptions: Indocin is more likely to cause ulcers, Feldene causes more gastrointestinal problems in people over age 60, and phenylbutazone is the most toxic (and is therefore rarely prescribed).

Be sure to ask your doctor to explain any side effects you might expect, and how best to cope with them. Bear in mind that you'll need to take most NSAIDs for up to six weeks to receive the maximum effect.

Acetylsalicylic acid. Otherwise known as aspirin, this is the least expensive NSAID. As it may cause ulcers, regular use may lead to bleeding. Enteric-coated products pass through the stomach first and then dissolve in the intestine, which lessens the risk of stomach problems. (Children should only be given aspirin substitutes such as acetaminophen, however. This is to avoid Reye's syndrome, a serious complication aspirin can cause.)

Nonacetylated salicylates: This group includes *choline magnesium trisalicylate (Trilisate)* and *salsalate (Disalcid, Salsitab)*. Generally, these do not damage the stomach lining and there's less chance of bleeding problems. They're used by people at risk for ulcers or gastrointestinal bleeding and may be good for those with impaired kidney function or who take diuretics. They may be less effective at relieving pain than the other NSAIDs, however.

Fenamate: This includes *meclofenamate sodium (Meclomen)*. It's effective for osteoarthritis and rheumatoid arthritis. Unfortunately, fenamate can cause bowel irritation and severe diarrhea. It's not recommended for children.

Idole-indene acetic acid derivatives. These include:
Diclofenac sodium (Voltaren). Spreading the tablets out throughout the day may lessen the chance of stomach irritation.
Etodolac (Lodine). Etodolac is more effective for treating osteoarthritis than rheumatoid arthritis.
Indomethacin (Indocin). Indomethacin is the most effective medicine for ankylosing spondylitis and severe osteoarthritis of the hip, and it is very effective in relieving acute gout. Although it works as well as other NSAIDs for rheumatoid arthritis, Indomethacin does cause more gastrointestinal and some central nervous system side effects, including

headache and sometimes forgetfulness or convulsions.
Sulindac (Clinoril). Possibly less likely to produce renal (kidney) side effects, sulindac can cause gastrointestinal irritation, headache, and rash.
Tolmetin sodium (Tolectin). Tolmetin is useful for osteoarthritis of the hip. Its side effects can include nausea, heartburn, indigestion and sometimes fluid retention.

Keto-naphthylalkanone. *Nabumetone (Relafen)* causes fewer minor stomach ulcers than most other NSAIDs and apparently doesn't damage the kidneys.

Phenylbutazone. This is one of the strongest NSAIDs and is usually advisable only for short-term use, due to bone marrow toxicity. It's used mostly for severe attacks in the hip and knee when other treatments don't help.

Propionic acid derivatives. Several of these are available both over the counter (OTC) and by prescription.
Fenoprofen calcium (Nalfon). Fenoprofen is the only NSAID that you should not take with food. Side effects may include kidney disease.
Ibuprofen (Advil, Motrin, Nuprin). In a few people this drug causes headache, fever, and a stiff neck. Dosages of OTC ibuprofen high enough to act as an NSAID may require many tablets daily. It may be easier and cheaper to take a prescription-strength version.
Ketoprofen (Actron, Orudis). Ketoprofen has been useful for osteoarthritis of the hip.
Naproxen (Naprosyn) and naproxen sodium (Anaprox, Aleve). Naproxen packs more punch per tablet, so you don't have to take as many pills as with other similar medications. (Other drugs, too, offer fewer doses, including Day-Pro, Voltaren, Clinoril, Relafen, and Feldene.)

CHAPTER 7

What if You Have Other Types of Arthritis?

While osteoarthritis and rheumatoid arthritis are by far the most common types of arthritis, there are many more. There is a mind-boggling array of more than 100 kinds of arthritis, including other joint conditions with similar symptoms. Not all of these are technically arthritis, but they sure feel like it.

When 69-year-old Ray got a pain in his right shoulder, for example, he thought the problem was osteoarthritis. He figured he'd just take Advil for a day or two and then his shoulder would be fine. What Ray didn't consider was that he had spent the last three days painting his living and dining rooms, and that activity had caused bursitis, not osteoarthritis.

For ease of reference, we've presented these other problems alphabetically.

BURSITIS AND TENDINITIS

Your body has about 150 bursae, small liquid-filled sacs that cushion muscles and tendons as they move within the body. Think of them as tiny balloons filled with something like mineral oil. When they're injured, from a blow, a fall, or just too much constant pressure, they fill with even more fluid and swell painfully. This is called bursitis, which just means swollen bursae.

Kneeling too long can bring on bursitis, whether you're scrubbing the floor or roofing a house. You can get it in your elbow, from a bump or from leaning it too long on a desk or table. Badly fitting or poorly designed shoes can cause bursitis in the hips or even bunions, bursitis in your toes. And, unfortunately, if you have painful arthritis, trying to compensate for sore joints by favoring one limb or moving awkwardly can irritate your bursae. Occasionally, bursitis is caused by an infection or by tendinitis.

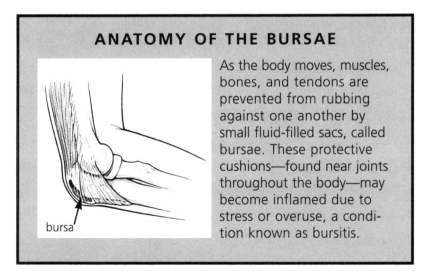

ANATOMY OF THE BURSAE

As the body moves, muscles, bones, and tendons are prevented from rubbing against one another by small fluid-filled sacs, called bursae. These protective cushions—found near joints throughout the body—may become inflamed due to stress or overuse, a condition known as bursitis.

bursa

Tendons are bands of tissue that connect your muscles to your bones. Tendinitis, or swollen tendon, is caused by stress on a tendon, or even a tear. You can get it in the heel, upper arm, elbow, wrist, hand, or hip. Because tendons and bursae are so close together, when tendons swell they can put pressure on the bursae, so you may often have both conditions at the same time, particularly in the shoulder. Doctors frequently diagnose the uncomfortable combo as "bursitis-tendinitis."

Symptoms. You may have dull pain around a joint that gets worse with movement and awakens you at night. The area may be swollen and warm when you touch it, and it will be red if the bursa is infected.

Diagnosis. This is based partly on your symptoms and on an examination of your joints and the tissues around them. Your doctor will ask questions: When did the pain start? What makes it worse? Have you had an injury? Your doctor will also examine you, which will usually allow her to know whether you have bursitis-tendinitis or arthritis. Occasionally, X-rays are also needed. Although bursitis isn't visible on X-rays, your doctor may have them taken to rule out other problems such as inflamed joints. And because infection is sometimes the cause, your doctor may remove some fluid from the bursa to check for a telltale high white blood cell count.

Prevention. The best way to prevent bursitis (and tendinitis as well) is to stay in shape, because then you're less likely to be injured from overuse. Also, stop activities when you feel pain. Avoid reaching overhead for long periods or moving your shoulder repeatedly such as in nonstop vacuuming. Take breaks, and stretch a bit. Use knee pads when roofing, gardening, or scrubbing floors; toss out shoes that are too tight or have well-worn heels; use shoe lifts or specially made shoes if one leg is longer than the other. Don't grip items too tightly. Tools or kitchen utensils with large handles, such as the ones designed for use with rheumatoid arthritis, will help keep you from squeezing too hard. Use your entire arm instead of your wrist whenever possible, whether you're hitting a tennis stroke or pushing open a door.

Treatment. The best news is that you can usually treat bursitis at home. Your primary treatments are rest and ice. Of course, first stop the activity that hurts, and then apply ice packs for 20 minutes every hour or two that you're awake. After 48 hours, switch to heat, such as a warm bath or a hot compress, for pain relief. You may want to take aspirin or an NSAID such as ibuprofen. After the pain lets up a bit, it's time to do some gentle stretching. Someone may sympathetically offer to massage the painful area for you, but just say no—this would make your bursitis worse. If you're in severe pain or still feel no relief in four days, see your doctor. Your doctor may inject cortisone into the bursa or remove fluid with a needle to check for infection. Very rarely, in extreme cases, the bursa may be surgically removed.

FIBROMYALGIA

Anna Sonnerup was a champion biathlete, a star of the demanding sport that combines cross-country skiing and target shooting. She was considered a shoo-in for the Olympics, but shortly before the trials she began to experience inexplicable periods of fatigue and weakness. They seemed to come and go. Then shockingly, at the preliminary trials she failed to qualify. What kept her from reaching the Olympics? It turned out that she had fibromyalgia, a disease predominated by muscle pain.

Next to osteoarthritis, fibromyalgia is probably the most common rheumatic problem. Found in women more often than men, it usually occurs between the ages of 20 and 50 and may affect as many as 2 percent of Americans. Fibromyalgia triggers pain in muscles, tendons, and ligaments rather than in the joints. Though it doesn't deform joints or limbs, it does cause pain and fatigue. Often, it causes depression, particularly because of the frustrating symptoms, but also because the condition is difficult to diagnose and poorly understood. Some researchers think it's caused by small traumas to the muscles—which may occur after flu or extreme physical or emotional stress—that decrease the blood flow. Others believe that the root of the disease is a sleep disorder that often occurs simultaneously. For some reason, in people with fibromyalgia, the deepest and most restful cycle of sleep is interrupted, although they may not be aware of it. Significantly, even healthy people showed symptoms of fibromyalgia when they were deprived of this type of sleep.

Symptoms. These include pain and stiffness, often in the whole body, but particularly in the neck, shoulders, hips, and lower back. People with fibromyalgia often complain of severe fatigue and feeling tired even after sleeping and may report other problems as well. Here's a breakdown of symptoms and how many people feel them:

+ Temporary numbness or tingling (called paresthesia)— 60 percent
+ Headaches—50 percent
+ Irritable bowel syndrome or abdominal pain, constipation, or diarrhea—30 to 50 percent
+ Sleep disorders, including apnea (when you stop breathing during sleep), and restless leg movements— 75 percent
+ Among women, pain during menstruation—40 percent
+ Depression—20 to 30 percent
+ Anxiety—50 percent

Diagnosis. This can be difficult. Your doctor will consider your symptoms and may run lab tests to check for conditions such as thyroid disease, rheumatoid arthritis, lupus, and polymyalgia rheumatica. Some people may have more than one condition: One in 10 people with rheumatoid arthritis, for example, also has fibromyalgia. And there's no simple blood test or X-ray evidence to confirm the disease. Since 1990, however, two specific guidelines for diagnosing this disorder have been used:

- Pain on both sides of the body for at least three months
- Pressure applied to at least 11 of 18 trigger points all over the body produces pain, often severe

Treatment. In treating fibromyalgia, your doctor has two primary goals: to ease your pain and help you sleep better. Here's how to achieve them.

Exercise. When you're suffering from fibromyalgia, you're tired and achy, and the last thing in the world you want to do is zip around the block. Crawling into bed feels more like it. But this lack of activity actually makes things worse, because muscles that aren't in shape feel pain more sharply. If you've been inactive, you need to start exercising again slowly, with as little as 10 minutes of daily walking. Every week, increase your time by 5 minutes until you're up to 30 to 40 minutes of exercise daily. If walking is too painful, try a non-weight-bearing activity such as swimming or bike riding. And remember that although it may be hard to believe right now, soon your workouts will make you feel better. Studies confirm that exercise can ease the pain and fatigue of fibromyalgia.

Change your sleep patterns. Generally, people with fibromyalgia don't have trouble falling asleep—they just don't rest well while they're sleeping. To help improve the quality of your sleep, go to bed and get up at the same time every day, even if it means getting up early on weekends. Forgo daytime naps, and avoid alcohol or caffeine in the evenings. (Drinks containing caffeine include cola drinks and other sodas such as Mountain Dew. Check the label if you're not sure if a beverage contains caffeine.) And sleeping pills are not a good idea. They may make things worse by interfering with the deep stages of sleep you need.

Start physical therapy. Your doctor may refer you to a physical therapist when you have painful flare-ups or when you need to build up an exercise program. A physical therapist can gently stretch your muscles after spraying the area with a solution that deadens the pain.

Learn proper body mechanics. Sometimes your job or a sport involves repetitive motions, and limiting or eliminating certain movements can reduce flare-ups. You can also work on your posture and learn to do certain tasks in a more mechanically "correct" fashion, such as changing how you grip your tennis racket or sitting in a different position at your computer. An occupational or physical therapist may offer valuable suggestions.

Consider medication. Fibromyalgia doesn't involve inflammation or swelling, so corticosteroids or high-dose NSAIDs won't help. You may, however, use acetaminophen (Tylenol) or over-the-counter low-dose NSAIDs such as aspirin, ibuprofen, or naproxen. Your doctor may prescribe low doses of antidepressants such as amitriptyline (Elavil) or nortriptyline (Pamelor), plus the muscle relaxant cyclobenzaprine, to help you sleep. Another helpful option is antidepressants such as fluoxetine (Prozac) or sertraline (Zoloft), which help block pain and restore normal sleep. One study found that people who took the antidepressant fluoxetine or amitriptyline slept better and felt less pain after taking the drug for six weeks. The two antidepressants together were twice as effective. Finding the right dose may take some time, however, and the effect is not immediate, so don't give up.

GOUT AND PSEUDOGOUT

If you've seen the old movie *Little Lord Fauntleroy*, or read the beloved children's book by Frances Hodgson

Burnett, you may remember the grumpy old grandfather, who often bellowed with pain because of his gouty big toe, and how his housekeeper scolded him about eating too many rich foods. She was right.

Eating foods such as liver, anchovies, and kidneys can contribute to or cause gout. These rich foods are high in purines, substances your body can change to uric acid. But we also produce uric acid in our bodies, and some people just produce too much.

When there's too much uric acid, some of it forms crystals in the joint and the joint lining (synovial membrane). Deposited calcium crystals in a joint cause a similar problem, pseudogout, which means false gout. Pseudogout usually involves the large joints, such as the wrists and knees and not the foot.

There are two types of gout: inherited, or primary, and secondary gout. In primary gout, the body simply produces too much uric acid, or you don't excrete as much in your urine as is normal. With secondary gout, there is too much uric acid in your blood either because you take diuretics (drugs that encourage urination) or because your kidneys are failing. Secondary gout can also result from chemotherapy treatment for cancer or from a disease such as leukemia that results in the breakdown of red blood cells. Most victims of gout are men over 40.

Symptoms. Unfortunately, gout attacks don't give you much warning. They often occur at night, and they hit fast. Three times out of four, they will strike the big toe with excruciating pain. The pain will gradually diminish over a one- to two-week period. You may not have another attack for months or years, but usually they begin to occur more frequently. Gout can affect the feet, knees, and elbows.

Diagnosis. Your doctor will suspect gout from the swelling, tenderness, and redness of your joints and from your other symptoms. Blood tests will usually show high uric acid. You may also have small lumps under the skin, often in the cartilage of your ear, caused by uric acid accumulation. If your doctor just isn't sure it's gout, he may aspirate, or draw fluid from, the joint to look for uric acid crystals. Occasionally, the doctor may give you a test dose of colchicine, a drug that can ease gout pain if given within 48 hours of an attack but won't work well on other types of arthritis. Later in the disease, X-rays can show bone damage caused by gout. (Pseudogout can also be diagnosed by calcium buildup in cartilage visible on X-rays and by the presence of calcium crystals in the joint fluid.)

Prevention. First, gout-proof your diet. High-purine foods, which include sardines, anchovies, sweetbreads, brains, kidney, and liver, are engraved invitations to a gout attack. But overweight itself is also a cause of gout. So if you're too heavy, adopt a commonsense, gradual weight loss plan. (But do it slowly and sensibly and never by fasting. Ironically, if you drop pounds too quickly, that can trigger gout attacks, too.) Be sure to drink plenty of water, and especially avoid alcohol, which not only is high in purines, but also prevents you from eliminating them through your urine.

You'll want to review your medications with your doctor if you are prone to gout. If you are taking the blood pressure medication hydrochlorothiazide (Esidrix, HydroDIURIL) or the diuretic, or "fluid pill," furosemide (Lasix), your doctor will want to switch you to different medicines. Niacin, sometimes prescribed to lower cholesterol, and daily aspirin can also cause problems. All of these drugs decrease the amount of uric acid that your kidneys can eliminate. Your doctor can steer you toward alternative drugs that won't encourage gout.

Finally, be aware that gout may flare up whenever you are admitted to the hospital, whether for surgery or a medical reason. It's not quite fair to discuss this under "Prevention," because if you could avoid injury or hospitalization, of course you would. But either event can raise your risk of gout. Make sure all your doctors know you're prone to gout problems if you're in the hospital or need surgery.

Treatment. Generally, it's best to stay in bed for 24 hours after a gout attack, because moving around can cause swelling and trigger another. A variety of medicines will help. Pseudogout is treated with aspirin or other NSAIDs. Primary and secondary gout are essentially treated in two stages. First, for an acute attack, your doctor may prescribe NSAIDs for the inflammation and pain or corticosteroids if NSAIDs are troublesome for you. In some cases your doctor may inject a drug called ketorolac (Toradol) into a muscle for pain. Or she may use indomethacin if you're having an acute attack. Sometimes corticosteroids are injected or fluid is drained from the joint to ease pain. Although a drug called colchicine was once widely prescribed for gout attacks, it's used less often today, because it is effective only at doses high enough to also cause diarrhea. Warning: If you take diuretics or low-dose aspirin for gout, you'll actually make things worse, as these drugs prevent your kidneys from excreting uric acid.

Then, after the attack subsides, your doctor will determine whether your uric acid levels need to be lowered by medication. Medications that lower uric acid levels do so in two ways. Drugs called uricosuric agents, such as probenecid and sulfinpyrazone, increase the amount of uric acid your kidneys eliminate. Others, such as allopurinol, work by lowering the amount of uric acid your body produces. You can't take uricosuric agents, however, if you have kidney problems. And, because gout medicines can interact with other drugs, be sure your doctor is aware of all the drugs you are taking.

One particularly dangerous interaction happens when allopurinol is mixed with azathioprine (or Imuran), an immunosuppressive drug sometimes prescribed for rheumatoid arthritis. (For more on Imuran, see chapter 6.) The problem? Allopurinol can make the effect of Imuran from 3 to 10 times stronger.

JUVENILE RHEUMATOID ARTHRITIS

Just as it sounds, juvenile rheumatoid arthritis attacks children, usually before age 17. About 200,000 children in the United States have this disease, which can range from mild to severe enough to cause serious complications. This disease does sometimes result in permanent joint damage or cause other problems because it can make children's bones grow at different rates. Although juvenile rheumatoid arthritis resembles the adult variety, thankfully it often goes away as the child matures into adulthood.

There are three types:

Pauciarticular—Affects four or fewer joints.

Polyarticular—Usually affects more than four joints. Resembles rheumatoid arthritis and has much the same prognosis.

Systemic onset (Still's disease)—High fevers; affects internal organs as well as joints. Also called febrile juvenile arthritis.

Symptoms. Most children with juvenile rheumatoid arthritis have warm, swollen, and painful joints. Parents may notice that a young child has begun to limp (because of knee or hip arthritis). The child often has less energy and may lose weight or stop growing. Fever is common, especially in Still's disease.

Diagnosis. As each type of juvenile rheumatoid arthritis has different symptoms, there's no single test for diagnosis. In general, the doctor will look for joint swelling, eye problems, and rashes and will examine X-rays and possibly synovial fluid.

Treatment. Generally, treatment includes anti-inflammatory drugs such as aspirin, range-of-motion exercises, splints, and bed rest. Surgery is sometimes needed to repair damaged joints, but it's often best to wait until adulthood when the disease has run its course. Regular eye exams are important because juvenile rheumatoid arthritis can cause eye inflammation, which can damage vision if not diagnosed and treated.

LUPUS

This oddly named disease, also called systemic lupus erythematosus (or SLE), strikes mainly women between the ages of 15 and 40. Eighty-five percent of the sufferers are female, and women of African descent are three times more likely to be affected than white women. If one identical twin is affected, the other is more vulnerable, and this and other factors suggest a genetic link. The causes, however, are not clearly understood.

Lupus is an autoimmune disease, like rheumatoid arthritis, in which the body "attacks" itself for some reason. And sometimes drugs you are taking for other problems may cause lupus symptoms. These include chlorpromazine (Thorazine), hydralazine (Apresoline), isoniazid (Laniazid, Nydrazid), methyldopa (Aldomet), procainamide (Pronestyl), and quinidine (Quinidex, Cardioquin).

The most common symptom is joint pain, which affects 9 of 10 people with lupus. In extreme cases, the lung lining, kidneys, heart, or brain can also become inflamed, and lupus may even be fatal. The severity of the disease varies greatly from person to person, however. Some cases are relatively harmless, some are severe, and sometimes lupus disappears and reappears without warning.

THE RISKS OF PREGNANCY WITH LUPUS

If you have lupus, being pregnant can put you at increased risk for many problems. These include:

- Toxemia, which can cause high blood pressure, retention of fluid, and seizures
- Spontaneous abortion
- Stillbirth
- Neonatal lupus, a rare condition that can cause a rash in newborns and sometimes a congenital heart defect called heart block
- Slowed growth of the developing baby

Your doctor should monitor your pregnancy closely and do specific blood work such as the anti-Ro and anti-La antibody tests. These antibodies increase the chance of having a baby with congenital heart block. The diagnosis of heart block is made by an echocardiogram and electrocardiogram (EKG) of the baby's heart. If you have kidney problems, your doctor will also keep a close watch on how your kidneys are working.

Even with milder cases, lupus may hit hard emotionally, because the necessary medications may change your body and your appearance. And that can be hard to handle. You may find you need to go through a grieving process over these changes before you begin to feel better about coping with the disease.

Symptoms. While aching joints are the most common symptom, fever and rashes are also common. Around half of lupus sufferers have a distinctive butterfly-shaped rash across the cheeks and nose, which may be triggered by exposure to the sun. Other symptoms include fatigue, weight loss, lethargy, and lack of appetite, although you may have relatively harmless lupus that requires little or no treatment. Loss of hair is common, and some people may develop sores or hives. Because there may be inflammation or swelling of the lining around the heart, lungs, or abdomen, it can hurt when you breathe deeply. Also, in those with an inflamed heart lining, heart failure can occur if the inflammation is not treated. You may develop eye problems including conjunctivitis, sensitivity to light, and blurred vision. Some people with lupus have colon problems or neurologic problems such as psychosis, seizures, strokes, and hallucinations.

Diagnosis. Because lupus can be difficult to diagnose, you may need to see a rheumatologist or other doctor who specializes in diagnosing and treating rheumatic diseases. Your doctor will take a blood test to determine if you have antinuclear antibodies, which almost always indicate lupus (although the test must be interpreted cautiously, as 1 to 5 percent of people without lupus also will have these antibodies). Other tests include blood count, to check for lowered hemoglobin, white blood cells and platelets; anti-DNA; anti-Sm; urinalysis; and kidney function tests. (For a review of these tests and what they reveal, see chapter 2.) If you meet 4 or more of 11 criteria that include rashes, sensitivity to light, ulcers in the mouth, and arthritis, it's likely to be lupus.

Treatment. Because lupus can affect different parts of your body and can strike with varying degrees of severity, treatment varies. You may have relatively harmless lupus that requires little or no treatment. You may simply need to protect your skin carefully from the sun, or use topical corticosteroids for skin problems. Rest and NSAIDs may be all you need to ease your joints. Eating a low-salt, low-fat diet will help, too. And here's your motivation to quit smoking: It's especially harmful because smoke increases the swelling in blood vessels affected by lupus. Finally, exercise regularly so your joints will keep working.

If you have rashes or more severe joint problems, you may require antimalarials or corticosteroids, and your doctor will likely prescribe steroids if the lupus has spread to the heart, lungs, or kidneys. Your doctor may also prescribe antimalarials or immunosuppressive drugs to help fight the inflammation.

LYME DISEASE

This disease that's gotten such big coverage results from the bite of a tiny deer tick, an insect about the size of a pinhead. Named after the Connecticut town where it was first documented, Lyme disease is prevalent in northern California, Wisconsin, Minnesota, and Pennsylvania and has been found in almost every state. Undiagnosed, it can result in crippling arthritis or nerve or heart problems. Prompt treatment, however, can keep arthritis and other problems from occurring at all.

Symptoms. Because the tick is so small, you likely won't see it. One possible warning sign is a circular rash, which shows up a few days or as long as a month after the bite. Most Lyme rashes resemble a red ring with a clear center and may continue to get bigger and bigger. But one out of three people with Lyme disease doesn't get the rash, so you can't count on this to alert you.

In the early stages, you may think you have the flu. You may have chills, fever, headaches, a stiff neck, swollen lymph nodes, fatigue, muscle aches, and joint pain. (But unlike most flu, you'll likely have these symptoms in spring and summer, when ticks are the most common.)

If arthritis does develop, the pain differs from most other types of arthritis because it seems to travel from joint to joint: You may feel it in your knee one week and in your elbow another. The arthritis may be intermittent at first or can be ongoing and disabling, often in the knees. Weeks or

years later, untreated Lyme causes arthritis of one joint—
usually the knee. Later symptoms can also include severe
headache and fatigue, drooping of your facial muscles, pain,
and numbness. If the disease isn't treated, it can also cause
heart problems, such as a slow or irregular heartbeat.

WHEN TO RUSH TO THE DOCTOR: INFECTIOUS ARTHRITIS

Sometimes joints become infected by a virus, bacterium,
or fungus that spreads through the blood. Warning signs
include the following:

- You feel pain and stiffness in one joint.
- The area around the joint is warm and red.
- You have chills and fever and feel weak.

If you have these symptoms, you need to be seen by a
doctor immediately.

Types of infectious arthritis include:

Lyme. Caused by bacteria transmitted by the bite of an
infected tick; produces fever, flu-like symptoms, and sometimes a round bull's-eye rash, followed by arthritis.

Gonococcal. Caused by the bacteria associated with the
sexually transmitted disease gonorrhea; produces sudden
joint pain that moves from joint to joint.

Rheumatic fever. Caused by streptococcal infection;
begins with a fever and throat infection. Untreated, it can
eventually damage the heart.

Other types of infectious arthritis result from infections
caused by bacteria (staphylococcal or tuberculous), plus relatively rare forms caused by fungi and viruses. Except for
those types caused by viruses, they are all treated with
antibiotics, and you may need to have joints drained with
a needle or have damaged areas surgically removed. If the
arthritis is caused by a bacterial infection, however, the
antibiotic therapy will usually cure it.

Diagnosis. If you have symptoms that suggest Lyme disease, your doctor will run a blood test called the Lyme titer that shows antibodies to spirochetes, the bacteria that cause the problem. (An antibody is a protein your body uses to fight an invader.) Other tests used to detect Lyme include the IFA (indirect immunofluorescence assay) or ELISA (enzyme-linked immunosorbent assay), along with a test called the Western blot.

Prevention. The best prevention is to wear a hat, long sleeves, and long pants in wooded areas. After your outing, inspect yourself carefully, and remove any tick you find. You should remove a tick with tweezers, as near its head as possible, and without squeezing its body. If you see an odd, circular rash, visit your doctor.

Treatment. Prompt treatment with antibiotics can protect you from arthritis and other serious complications. If you already have developed Lyme arthritis, your doctor will still likely administer antibiotics, but also treat the arthritis just as she does other types of inflammatory diseases.

POLYMYALGIA RHEUMATICA AND GIANT CELL ARTERITIS

These two conditions are closely linked, and some doctors believe they are different aspects of the same disease. (Ten to 15 percent of people with polymyalgia rheumatica also have giant cell arteritis, and similarly, 40 percent of people with giant cell arteritis have polymyalgia rheumatica.)

Polymyalgia Rheumatica

This relatively "new" disease wasn't named until 1957, partly because it can be difficult to diagnose. But about 5 out of 1,000 people have it, most of them over 50. Twice as many women as men have polymyalgia rheumatica, and it's more common in white people than in people of African descent. The early symptoms are similar in many ways to those of rheumatoid arthritis: The linings of the shoulder joints (synovial tissues) are often inflamed, though the muscles are normal.

Symptoms. Morning pain and stiffness occur in the neck, hips, and shoulders, with pain felt on both sides of the body in the same places. Moving makes the muscle pain worse. You may be tired and lose weight without intending to. You may also have low fever, night sweats, and depression.

Diagnosis. Different doctors propose different methods for diagnosing polymyalgia rheumatica, as there is no single standard test. But they will take particular note if you are older than 50, have no rheumatoid factor and negative antinuclear antibodies, and are experiencing at least three of these symptoms:

- Pain in the neck, shoulder, or hip
- Morning stiffness that lasts more than an hour
- A high sed rate, above 40 millimeters per hour (although about 13 percent will have a normal sed rate)
- A rapid response to a dose of prednisone (a corticosteroid)

Many people will have a sed rate above 100 millimeters per hour, plus mild anemia and a raised platelet count. One-third of people with polymyalgia rheumatica will have slightly abnormal liver function tests. Your doctor may run these tests: sed rate, complete blood count, thyroid function, chest X-ray, rheumatoid factor, synovial fluid test, a biochemical profile, and a few others.

Treatment. NSAIDs may help control symptoms for a few people with this disease, but corticosteroids are almost always necessary. Treatment usually continues for one to three years, but for some people it may take longer. Unfortunately, corticosteroids can have significant and serious side effects, including infections, broken bones due to osteoporosis, and difficulty in controlling diabetes and high blood pressure. Your doctor will monitor you to help offset these problems.

Giant Cell Arteritis

This disease, in which some blood vessels become inflamed, has a sometimes puzzling link with polymyalgia rheumatica. In Scandinavia, nearly half the time they occur together; in the northern United States, they occur together in 20 people out of 100. Oddly, though, both diseases occur together only a tiny percentage of the time in Israel. Giant cell arteritis can appear before, during, or after polymyalgia rheumatica. As with polymyalgia rheumatica, those affected are mostly white females over the age of 50, and there's probably a genetic link. Three times as many women as men have it.

The major difference is that unlike polymyalgia rheumatica, giant cell arteritis can potentially cause blindness. Also, although polymyalgia rheumatica responds to low-dose prednisone (10 to 20 milligrams per day), giant cell arteritis requires a higher dose of 40 to 60 milligrams daily.

Symptoms. They can be flu-like, but with no apparent virus. Symptoms include fatigue, severe headaches, difficulty hearing, pain in the joints, and tender scalp. Blurry or double vision, and sometimes even loss of vision, can develop. Some sufferers will have thick, tender arteries with weak pulses. If untreated, giant cell arteritis can lead to blindness, stroke, or heart attack.

Diagnosis. Tests your doctor is likely to run are the same as for polymyalgia rheumatica: sed rate, complete blood count, and liver function tests. Sed rate may be higher than normal. Your doctor will also probably do a temporal artery biopsy, a minor operation that involves taking a very small piece of the artery from your temple, in front of your ear, and examining it under a microscope. However, inflammation in this artery doesn't show up in 10 to 20 percent of people with this disease.

Treatment. High doses of corticosteroids are the standard treatment. Dramatic improvement is usually seen within a few days.

SJÖGREN'S SYNDROME

This disease is often an unwelcome companion to rheumatoid arthritis or other rheumatic diseases, but it can also appear on its own. Ninety percent of people with Sjögren's syndrome are women, and their average age is 50. Fortunately, it progresses slowly, and doesn't fully develop for as long as 10 years after it starts. Sjögren's is an autoimmune condition in which immune cells attack three glands in your body. Called exocrine glands, they normally produce saliva, sweat, and tears. With Sjögren's, they go haywire and don't work as they should, thus drying out your eyes, mouth, and other areas.

Symptoms. You may feel as if you have something like a grain of sand stuck in your eye, and your eyes may itch and burn. They also may be more sensitive to light. You may have mouth troubles, too: difficulty chewing and swallowing dry foods, small sores on your tongue or lips, and a burning sensation. Food may taste different than it used to. And, because you produce less saliva, which normally helps clean debris from your mouth, you'll be more prone to cavities.

Diagnosis. Your doctor will suspect Sjögren's syndrome because of your primary symptoms: dry eyes and mouth. She will do some detective work, such as checking your medications and asking you about over-the-counter products you may have been using, to find out if there's another likely cause of your symptoms. She may then run a test called the Schirmer test to check how much tears and saliva you produce. Seven of 10 people with Sjögren's will have rheumatoid factor, so she'll probably test for that and possibly other antibodies as well. Blood tests may also reveal mild anemia and a low number of cells called leukocytes in the blood.

Treatment. The usual approach is to try to replace the fluids you are lacking, primarily by using artificial tears for your dry eyes. To ease your dry mouth, your doctor will recommend drinking plenty of water, avoiding alcohol, and possibly switching from medications that decrease saliva flow, such as some high blood pressure drugs and certain antidepressants. You'll need more frequent dental checkups and will need to avoid the sugary foods that cause cavities. You may also need moisturizing cream for your skin.

INFLAMMATORY ARTHRITIS AND THE SPINE

The following types of inflammatory arthritis can all affect the spine, and they also have a genetic link. It's important to be aware that a genetic link does not mean that if you have one of these diseases you'll automatically give it to your children, however. A person can have the gene for a particular type of arthritis and never develop any signs of arthritis at all.

Ankylosing spondylitis. "Ankylosing" means rigid, "spondyl" means spine, and "itis" means inflamed, which pretty well describes this disease. It makes hips, shoulders, ribs, back, and neck stiff and sore and can cause a stiff, inflexible backbone. If you have a relative with ankylosing spondylitis, you have an increased risk. Men get it more often than women, usually during their 30s. It often goes undiagnosed but can cause serious damage. If a parent has ankylosing spondylitis, the child has a one in two to one in four chance of getting the gene. If you have inherited the gene, then you have a one in ten chance of developing the disease.

Ankylosing spondylitis comes on gradually and, if not treated, eventually can "fuse" the entire spine. Symptoms include a chronic low backache; gradually worsening inability to move the back and expand the chest fully when breathing; X-ray changes in sacroiliac joints in the spine; high sed rate; and negative rheumatoid factor. A test for the antigen HLA-B27 is usually positive. Treatment includes anti-inflammatories and exercise, including range-of-motion and stretching. Because it can affect the rib cage and hence limit your breathing, it's important to maintain good posture. It's also important to avoid using more than one pillow at night. Sleeping with your head propped up increases the possibility of causing the neck, already affected by the disease, to become permanently bent. Your doctor will also advise you to quit smoking and may prescribe NSAIDs, particularly indomethacin.

Arthritis of inflammatory bowel disease. Inflammatory bowel disease includes intestinal problems such as ulcerative colitis and Crohn's disease. About 10 percent of people with ulcerative colitis and 20 percent of those with Crohn's disease wind up with one of two kinds of associated arthritis. One is a form of spinal arthritis that appears similar to ankylosing spondylitis. The other causes mostly morning pain and stiffness in the hands, knees, and elbows. Treatment is simply anti-inflammatories and better control of the bowel disease itself.

Psoriatic arthritis. You may know someone with psoriasis, a skin condition that results in swollen, red, and often scaly skin. One person in 10 with psoriasis will also get psoriatic arthritis. It will likely cause pain in the joints, but fortunately, it's not usually disabling. Treatment includes anti-inflammatories such as aspirin and sometimes other drugs and range-of-motion exercises. Psoriatic arthritis usually does not affect the same parts on both sides of the body. In severe cases, fingers and toes may swell enough to resemble sausages. Tests will show that rheumatoid factor is negative, sed rate is high, and uric acid may be up. X-rays are useful, as they can show your doctor areas of joint or bone damage.

Reiter's syndrome. Found mostly in young white men, this type of arthritis occurs as a reaction either to certain sexually transmitted infections, particularly urethritis and dysentery, or to a gastrointestinal infection that produces severe diarrhea. Reiter's syndrome is also called reactive arthritis, because joints are reacting to the infection in the body by becoming inflamed.

The symptoms usually appear one to four weeks after a sexually transmitted genital or urinary tract infection (usually accompanied by frequent, burning urination) or gastrointestinal problem. A knee, ankle, or foot on one side may become tender or swollen. Fever and weight loss are common. There may be pain in the ribs, spine and lower back, and heel and Achilles tendon (places where ligaments attach to the bone). Other symptoms may include swollen, reddened eyes, a rash, and inflammation of the urethra, the small tube through which you urinate.

The doctor will diagnose Reiter's by examining you, performing blood tests, and taking X-rays, if there appear to be bone changes around the sacroiliac joint of the spine. In some cases of Reiter's, antibiotics may be helpful. Otherwise, treatment usually includes rest, NSAIDs for pain, and sometimes corticosteroids for skin problems.

CHAPTER 8

When Surgery Is Necessary

You exercise conscientiously and wisely; you choose your foods carefully and you've lost your excess weight. You have faithfully limited activity that would make your arthritis worse, and you and your doctor have explored many types of medication. But you're still in such pain that your lifestyle has dramatically changed.

Forty years ago, if you had severe osteoarthritis of the knee or hip, for example, you might easily have wound up bed-bound. Today, there's a far brighter future, thanks to remarkable surgical procedures that can leave you feeling like a new person. In most cases, people with arthritis for whom surgery is appropriate will find themselves dramatically improved.

So if your doctor says, "We'll need to consider surgery," the truth is those may be the most encouraging words you've heard yet.

Of course, it's natural to feel cautious about surgical procedures. Just as you shouldn't rule out surgery without considering it, neither do you want to leap into the operating room without considering the pros and cons. No two people are identical: A type of operation that works wonderfully for one may not be suitable for another. There are many possibilities, ranging from various types of joint replacements to a minor procedure that you can watch on a television screen while it's underway.

In most cases, surgery doesn't need to take place right away, so you'll have some time to consider your options, prepare for the operation, and plan for your recovery period afterward.

Here are the types of surgery available.

WHAT IS ARTHROSCOPY?

Arthroscopy may become your best friend. For some problems, this relatively quick and simple procedure can have you walking out of the hospital just a few hours after you limped in on crutches. Named after the clever instrument, arthroscopy is done using an arthroscope, a bundle of very thin, light-transmitting glass fibers inside a tube about the thickness of a pencil. It is attached to a small camera, which lets the surgeon see right inside your joint.

How is it done? This fascinating procedure can often be performed while you are awake, with just the area to be operated on numbed. In these cases, you can watch on a television monitor. If the procedure is to be done on your knee, you will likely receive an epidural anesthetic, a shot near your spine that anesthetizes you from the waist down. You'll have an intravenous line, and your heart rate and blood pressure will be monitored. An orthopedic surgeon will make a tiny cut, then insert the arthroscope into your joint. The surgeon can then use the tube to look around and see what the problem is or insert small surgical instruments through it to repair cartilage and remove loose pieces of bone, all the while watching the inside of your joint on the monitor.

Who gets it? Damage to cartilage or to bone (such as loose bone fragments) in a specific, localized area of a joint may qualify you for arthroscopy. The vast majority of these procedures are done for knees (around 85 percent), around 10 percent for shoulders, and around 5 percent for other joints. Arthroscopy is virtually never used for the hips.

What are the pros and cons? You don't have to stay in the hospital overnight, and you have only tiny incisions. Generally, the only possible complications are infections and some residual pain or stiffness. While this procedure can remove or smooth out damaged cartilage and remove bone bits, it cannot replace or actually repair your existing cartilage.

WHAT IS A SYNOVECTOMY?

Rheumatoid arthritis develops because of a diseased synovium, or joint-lining membrane, which releases substances that damage the cartilage, ligaments, tendons, and bone. A synovectomy is simply the removal of this membrane. Usually the joint surfaces are also smoothed in a procedure called debridement.

The problem with synovectomy is that the synovium often grows back and becomes inflamed again. This procedure should generally be considered only if you have severe joint pain that doesn't respond to medication.

How is it done? Your surgeon may advise regular surgery or may be able to perform arthroscopy using the tiny incisions that don't require general anesthesia. Rare cases call for radiation synovectomy, a procedure that destroys the synovium with a radioactive substance. Newer options still being investigated include laser synovectomy, which uses a laser to destroy the synovium through an arthroscope, and chemical synovectomy, in which chemical agents destroy the diseased synovium.

Who gets it? Synovectomy is most often recommended if you have severe rheumatoid arthritis that can't be controlled by medication. Some doctors believe these procedures should be done in the early stages of the disease; others believe they should be done after the disease has progressed; and still others don't believe in them at all. You'll want to discuss synovectomy thoroughly with your doctor and consider all possible options.

What are the pros and cons? With the removal of the synovium, pain and swelling decrease and the joint damage is halted. You may, however, feel stiffness in the joint afterward. And after several years, the synovium may grow back. Standard synovial surgery requires several months of recovery time, but if your procedure can be done by arthroscopy, you can recover in just a few weeks.

A LOOK AT JOINT REPLACEMENT

People whose joints are irreparably damaged by osteoarthritis may need joint replacement. In this procedure, which is also called arthroplasty, the surgeon removes the diseased or damaged pieces of bone and installs a synthetic substitute. Instead of bone, you'll have stainless steel; instead of cartilage, you'll have a durable plastic such as Teflon. The artificial joint is either attached with surgical cement or allowed to gradually attach itself as real bone grows into the joint.

While the surgery may sound somewhat drastic, it can make your life feel worth living again. To people who have been homebound, unable even to walk through the house without pain, it can seem like a miracle. About 150,000 people a year have joint replacements, most often due to arthritis, and hip replacements are the most common procedures. If you are substantially overweight, you may not be considered a good candidate, however, because the extra weight would put too much stress on the joint.

Hips and knees are both large joints and reasonably easy to replace. These surgeries are common, and the prognosis for recovery is excellent. One or two out of every 100 hip replacements "fail" because of infections or blood clots. Hips, a simple ball-and-socket arrangement, are the simplest to replace, while knees are a bit more complex. Look at your knee: It bends back, but side-to-side movement is limited. That makes it a fairly complicated hinge.

Although less common, artificial joints are also available for ankles, elbows, shoulders, and fingers. They aren't as advanced as artificial knees and hips, so they leave something to be desired. (In some cases, wrist or ankle joints may need to be fused rather than replaced; they will be inflexible, but because bone is no longer rubbing against bone, the pain will vanish.) Replacement of finger joints can relieve pain, improve appearance and some function, but the new fingers, of course, aren't nearly as good as the nonarthritic originals were. A relatively new implant for the wrist, which fuses an L-shaped metal plate to the finger and wrist bones, has worked for some people. In one study, it took about two and a half months for the implant to fuse to the bones, but afterward people could grip normally, had less pain and swelling, and found that their wrists were more stable than before the surgery.

Much progress has been made in replacement joints since the 1960s. These older joints would last only 10 to 15 years, while today's can last much longer. How long, of course, depends on how much stress the new joint is subjected to. Vigorous activity will wear it out more quickly.

A CLOSER LOOK AT HIPS AND KNEES

Two people with the same amount of joint damage and similar lifestyles can both have joint replacements. But one may declare the operation a success, and the other may be bitterly disappointed.

Part of what determines the success of your new joint is what you expect of it. While great advances have been

ARE YOU READY FOR A NEW JOINT?

Joint replacement is, of course, a surgical procedure, and doctors don't want to put you through it if it isn't necessary or the time isn't right. Even if your pain is severe, surgery may not be the only option. Sometimes losing weight or changing medicines can do the job quickly and much less traumatically. Other times exercises will help. Surgery is only for pain and disability that won't respond to other treatments.

Generally, however, if you meet these five criteria, you are likely to be helped most by joint replacement:

- Despite making changes in your lifestyle, such as losing weight and doing exercises, your arthritis is seriously affecting the quality of your life.
- Drug treatments are not helping enough.
- Your joint hurts so much that sometimes it wakes you up at night.
- You have so much pain that you can walk only about a block.
- Your X-rays show significant damage in the joint.

Your doctor may also consider other factors, such as any other condition you may have, including diabetes or heart disease, and the possible effect of surgery on those problems. And you may want to consider the cost of the procedure, the time required for recovery, and the expected benefits. Once you've explored all the options and ramifications, if you and your doctor decide that it's time to have a joint replaced, you can go into surgery knowing you've made the very best choice for you.

made with artificial limbs, futuristic replacements that look and work even better than the originals are still a long way off. Your new joint may work well, but it won't be the same as your "real" joint was when it was healthy.

And replacement joints, just like the originals, don't last forever. How long they last, just like the originals, can depend on how you treat them. Jogging, for example, is a lot tougher on a joint than bicycling or swimming.

Here are some more things to mull over.

Consider the true costs. If you've been putting off a hip replacement in the interests of saving money, think again. When a study compared the costs of having a hip replaced with not having it replaced—including such things as quality of life as well as life expectancy—it found that a hip replacement could save money. With a hip replacement, a 60-year-old woman could theoretically live alone and take care of herself for 20 years before needing help during her last two years of life. Without the hip replacement, that woman would likely need daily help for 15 years and then be bedridden for about eight years. And the long-term care she would require would cost twice as much as the surgery.

Kneecap replacement. Doctors have disagreed about whether it's necessary to replace part of your kneecap, a process called resurfacing, during a knee joint replacement. When 50 people with osteoarthritis in the knee had the resurfacing and 50 did not, the group without the kneecap resurfacing had less pain and better knee flexibility. Yet the only two people who had to have their surgeries repeated did not have their kneecaps resurfaced in the first procedure.

When two is better than one. If both your knees need replacing, you may want to consider having both done at once. It's generally cheaper, and you'll go through just one recovery period and spend less time overall in the hospital. One study found that if you have severe arthritis symptoms in that second knee, there's a good chance it will need replacing within the next decade. Of 185 people in the study, almost all with severe symptoms in one knee to be replaced required a second new knee within the decade.

(On the other hand, only 38 percent of those with only moderate symptoms in their "good" knee needed it replaced before a decade had passed.)

WHICH TYPE OF JOINT?

You may have hoped this would be easy—you just order up a new knee or hip, and in it goes. But it's not quite that simple. You and your doctor need to consider if you will have a cemented or uncemented joint and what type of knee prosthesis to use.

Cemented. Cemented is just like it sounds. Remember that tube of cement you used as a child to glue model airplanes together? It's not the same glue, of course, but the idea is the same: The new joint is actually glued to the bone. Your joint heals quickly, but about half the time, it will loosen or become unglued in 10 to 20 years. When this happens, you may need more surgery to reglue the joint, a procedure called a revision. Revisions are more complicated than the original surgery, as more bone must be cut away and the surgery takes longer.

Generally, the cemented joints are recommended for people over 65. One reason is that bones have grown thinner in many older people, and for these people a cemented joint may work better. But this is hardly a fixed rule. If you're a healthy, active 70-year-old, for instance, you probably have stronger bones than a sedentary person 20 years younger who already has osteoporosis, or thinning of the bones. (Osteoporosis is linked to a lack of calcium and vitamin D. It can be hereditary and is most common in postmenopausal women who do not take supplemental estrogen, although some men suffer osteoporosis as well.)

Uncemented. With uncemented joints, your existing bone actually grows right into the bumpy, sandpapery material of your new joint. It produces a tighter bond, but because it isn't initially fastened as tightly as cemented joints, it takes longer to heal. You should be prepared to spend more recovery time, perhaps three or more months on crutches, and postpone dancing that jig at your nephew's wedding.

Full or partial. Knees are complicated apparatuses, so surgeons have developed two options for knee replacements. Your knee has two compartments, inside and outside. A total (bicondylar) knee prosthesis replaces both compartments. It has two parts: the femoral part, a metal unit that fits on top of your femur bone, and a tibial part, a metal "tray" on a stem that's fastened to your tibia. After this procedure, you'll walk freely but be able to bend your new knee only 90 to 110 degrees, less than the 140 degrees of a natural knee.

A unicompartmental (unicondylar) knee prosthesis replaces only one compartment of the knee, either the inside or the outside one. An obvious benefit is that it's less extensive surgery and allows more knee flexibility than a total replacement. Doctors may recommend this for young, active people who will be more likely to wear out their prosthesis, thus minimizing the amount of later surgery they may need.

A LOOK AT OTHER PROCEDURES

Here's a rundown of other procedures your doctor may recommend.

Osteotomy. In Greek, this means bone cutting, and that's exactly what it is. Bone near a damaged joint, often the knee, is cut away and the rest of the bones are realigned, sometimes by removing or adding wedges of bone. Osteotomy particularly helps people with osteoarthritis whose cartilage has eroded unevenly, resulting in joints that don't line up right. This procedure can straighten out slight abnormalities that may have caused you to be a bit bow-legged or knock-kneed, for example. Good candidates are people with mild arthritis in just one compartment of the knee and those who are too young or otherwise not ready for joint replacement. Some researchers recommend an osteotomy for people who want to continue sports that involve running or jumping or a job that requires bending or lifting. In about six weeks, you'll be 80 percent recovered, and after six months, fully recovered. Of 34 men aged 60 and under who had osteotomies, 28 of them were happy with the surgery, and most could continue their previous activities, such as skiing and bicycling. After an average of seven years, 8 of the 34 required a second operation, mostly joint replacement.

Resection. This is a fancy word for removal of all or part of a bone, generally in the hands, wrists, elbows, ankles or toes. It can relieve pain in the feet, for example, when body weight is distributed unevenly and dislocated parts of the bones bear the brunt of the burden with each step. Usually people with rheumatoid arthritis can benefit from resection; recovery can take several weeks.

Arthrodesis. In this procedure, two bones are fused, or fastened together, permanently. This is used for unstable, painful joints that can't usually be replaced, such as in the wrists, feet, ankles, and thumbs, and occasionally for joints in the back or neck. In the knee, for example, the femur and tibia would be joined so that they basically become one bone. After arthrodesis, the joint cannot be moved, but it's more stable and you'll no longer feel pain. For several months after surgery, you'll have to wear a brace. That can place additional strain on adjoining joints, and once in a while joints become unfused. Arthrodesis is seldom chosen unless a joint replacement is impossible.

WHAT HAPPENS IN JOINT REPLACEMENT SURGERY

A total joint replacement, also called an arthroplasty, will substitute synthetic materials for the damaged bone surfaces in a joint. For example, in hip arthroplasty—the most common operation—a metal ball replaces the rounded head of the femur (thigh bone), while the pelvic socket, or acetabulum, is cleaned out and replaced with a metal cup lined with an extremely strong, high-grade plastic called polyethylene. The artificial components may be fastened

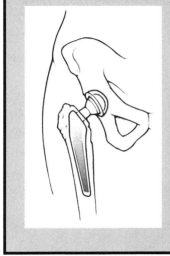

to the bone with cement, or they may be covered with a porous material that forms a firm attachment to the bone over time.

The metal and plastic implants used in arthroplasty glide over each other with very little friction, allowing for smooth, pain-free motion. While patients may experience some initial pain after the procedure—due to the movement of muscles during the surgery—most notice an immediate, dramatic decrease in pain.

THE NITTY GRITTY OF SURGERY

You and your doctor have determined that surgery is the best option for you. Now you need to find answers to some specific questions.

Who does it? The person who operates on you will generally be an orthopedic surgeon. Or sometimes you may need a hand surgeon who has also been trained in either orthopedic or plastic surgery. As with most things in life, practice makes perfect, so feel free to ask how often the doctor has done this operation. Often, a surgeon at a teaching hospital or joint center will have more procedures under his belt. And while your surgeon's skill is important, it's also crucial that you feel comfortable asking questions.

Select the hospital. Your options may be limited by where your chosen orthopedic surgeon operates, where you live, or where your health plan will allow you to go. If you have the luxury, however, you'll want to choose a hospital with a good general reputation that's also known for orthopedics.

What to expect afterward. Ask your doctor specifically what you'll be able to do after your successful surgery. It's crucial to tell the doctor exactly what activities you most enjoy or what your work involves, because the surgeon may use different techniques, depending on your goals. Whether or not you consider your procedure a success will partly depend on the expectations you carry into surgery. So if you want to be able to pole-vault after surgery, and it leaves you only able to walk and swim free of pain, you may be disappointed. But if you know ahead of time that pole-vaulting isn't realistic, you're more likely to be happy with the activities you can do.

Consider a second opinion. Your insurance may or may not pay for your visit to another doctor, but many people feel that it's a wise investment before you undertake a costly medical procedure. You need to make sure you're making the choice that's right for you.

Get the specifics. Take a notepad with a list of questions for your doctor. You'll want to know:

- Are there any alternatives to this type of surgery?
- What's involved in this operation? How long will it take?
- How long will I stay in the hospital?
- How much time is required for rehabilitation? Will I need physical therapy? In the hospital or at home?

- Will I need crutches or a walker while I recover?
- How much time will I have to take off from work?
- How many times have you done this procedure?
- What is the cost? (You'll have to ask your health insurance representative how much is covered by your insurance.)
- Is a blood transfusion necessary? Can I donate my own blood in advance?
- What after-surgery care will I need? Will I need home nursing, a physical therapist, an occupational therapist, or a nutritionist?

THINGS TO DO BEFORE YOU LEAVE HOME

You've weighed your options, discussed the procedure with your doctor, and your surgery date is reserved. Ready to go, right?

A little forethought can make things a whole lot easier during your hospital stay and when you come home. And sometimes it can help prevent some unpleasant surprises.

Here's a checklist.

Catch up on paperwork. This includes arranging for deposits of income and paying bills that will become due during your hospital stay and your first few weeks of recovery. And, not to borrow trouble, but if you're like most of us, you'll go into any operation with an easier mind if you've asked your lawyer to draw up a power of attorney and update your will if necessary.

Visit your dentist. You should have any necessary dental work done well before the operation. Bacteria from even a minor infection elsewhere in the body, like the mouth, can get into your bloodstream and travel to the joint. One thing you don't want is to have your new joint get infected, and this can happen if unfriendly bacteria start swimming around in your bloodstream. (If you need dental work after your joint replacement, your doctor may prescribe preventive antibiotics in advance for safety's sake. Be sure to check with your doctor before any dental work.)

Assess your surroundings. Look around at your home or office as though you're seeing it during your recovery period. If you'll be using crutches or a walker, how easy will it be to get around? Tidy up and move obstacles out of the way. If your bedroom is upstairs, consider lining up some helpers to set up a temporary downstairs bedroom and make it cheerful. Your friends will be just as happy to hold your hand in the living room. (You'll find some handy hints on rearranging things in chapter 9.)

Go shopping. Stock up on grocery staples and household items now. Prepare and freeze meals ahead of time. Now's the time to indulge in that novel you've been wanting to read or borrow stacks of videos from your neighbor. Your local library, besides lending books, probably also lends videos; update your library card and check things out ahead of time. If you have a computer and modem, often you can search the library catalogs and request titles you want and even renew items over the modem.

Pack with care. Be choosy about what to take with you to the hospital. Pack comfy pajamas and robe but not your favorites (there's a chance they'll get stained), nonslip slippers, an inexpensive watch or clock, magazines, and phone numbers of friends and relatives. Leave your valuables at home, but don't forget a favorite photo. A small inexpensive tape player with headphones can fill your mind with music.

HOW TO AVOID POCKETBOOK SHOCK

In these days of confusing and rapidly changing health insurance plans, you can't overdo the questions about what is and what is not covered.

Ask the hospital:

- Who are all the separate health care professionals I will receive a bill from? Often the surgeon, anesthesiologist, and physical therapist, for example, send a bill separate from the hospital's.

And ask your health insurance representative:

- Is this hospital a preferred or approved hospital? Which of my doctors are preferred? While your surgeon might be "preferred," your anesthesiologist might not be, which can make a big difference in how much money you have to shell out. It's best to know ahead of time.

- How long a hospital stay is allowed? You don't want to be arguing this while you're in the hospital and perhaps feeling bad. Get this spelled out ahead of time. Ask exactly what's required if your doctor feels you need more recovery time in the hospital than your health plan specifies.

- Precisely what after-surgery care is paid for? Your doctor may want you to work with a physical therapist, an occupational therapist, or a nutritionist. Find out if these are covered, and get names of preferred or approved ones.

- Are crutches, splints, or a walker paid for? If so, how do you get the claim forms? Do you need to purchase or rent these aids from a specific place?

- Is home health care paid for? If not, and your doctor recommends it, some communities offer home care for payment on a sliding scale, which means it's based on your ability to pay. You may need only a recommendation from your doctor.

Ask your company benefits administrator:

- Do I get disability pay from work, and how much is it and how long will it last?

WHAT TO EXPECT AFTER SURGERY

Right after a joint replacement, you're not going to feel ready for your tango lesson. The joint itself shouldn't pain you, but muscles moved around during the surgery will hurt. Depending on the nature of your surgery and your immediate postoperative condition, your doctor may provide oral painkillers ranging from Tylenol to codeine derivatives. On the first day after therapy, you may start passive exercises, with a therapist gently moving your limb. This will help strengthen the muscles around the new joint. On the second day, you'll probably be allowed to walk around, using a walker and later crutches. You'll feel pretty doddery, but hang in there; it gets better.

Though you'll be able to get around, take it easy for a while. Your joint won't be 100 percent healed for some time. So it's crucial to follow your doctor's directions carefully (and to ask questions if you're unsure of any specifics). With a hip replacement, you'll likely be 80 percent recovered after four weeks and completely recovered in six months. If your knee was replaced, it will take six weeks to reach that 80 percent mark, six months to be 90 percent recovered, and a full year before you're completely healed.

One important partner in your recovery will be a physical therapist, who will design a specific exercise program for you. The physical therapist will discuss the treatment plan with you and write out the entire program, including diagrams of how to do each exercise. She will also discuss how long you can expect your recovery to take and set both long- and short-term goals you should aim for.

You may be asked to do continuous passive motion (CPM). For a recovering knee, for example, you would sit while a device at the foot of your bed bends and straightens your leg continuously, several hours a day, while you watch

Oprah or read. Gradually, the movement will increase the range of motion in your joint. CPM, in combination with regular physical therapy, can help your joint recover faster and reduce swelling after the operation. Also, the cost of a CPM device is less than having a physical therapist do all of the work with you.

It's normal to grow impatient during the recovery period. It's easy to forget how bad things were *before* the surgery and why you had it in the first place. But the ultimate success of your new joint and your recovery depends partly on your commitment to take good care of yourself and your joint. A postsurgical joint will never be just like the original before the arthritis, but an operation can allow you to resume a more active and nearly pain-free life. Depending on your situation, you may have to walk briskly instead of run marathons or play volleyball instead of tackle football, but your life can still be vigorous and full.

QUESTIONS TO ASK YOUR DOCTOR BEFORE YOU LEAVE THE HOSPITAL

- When will I start physical therapy?
- How long should I stay in bed?
- How long should the joint be painful?
- How long can I expect my joint to last?
- Can I run, swim, or bicycle? How long and how fast?
- What activities or kinds of movement should I avoid?
- Are there special exercises I should do?

CHAPTER 9

Helping Yourself Live with Arthritis

You have arthritis. And until scientists have perfected modern-day miracles such as regrowing cartilage or being able to control our immune cells (they're working on it), arthritis can't be cured completely.

How frankly you face your arthritis, however, can make a huge difference in how you are able to cope with the problem and how much it affects the quality of your life.

You may need to be flexible and change how you do things. You may have to give up some activities and substitute others. And some people believe that your attitude can affect your immune system and how your body functions, so you may want to work on how you think about things as well. The bottom line? There are many, many ways to adapt and compensate so that arthritis has the least possible impact on how you live.

GIVE YOUR JOINTS A HELPING HAND

If you have rheumatoid arthritis, you're well aware that day-to-day activities can be very painful. Small helpful devices or gadgets designed to make it easier to grip or reach things can go a long way toward making your life more comfortable. Some aids, such as the ones listed subsequently, you can make on your own or buy at a drugstore.

One of the best places to find out about helpful devices such as these is the *Guide to Independent Living for People with Arthritis*. Produced by the Arthritis Foundation, this publication features just about every item imaginable. (To contact the foundation, call 800-283-7800 or go to your computer and look up *http://www.arthritis.org* on the Internet.)

Fatter handles. Getting a grip on small everyday items such as knives and potato peelers can be particularly painful. If you buy new ones, choose those with fat rubberized handles that are easy to grip. To convert your old ones, get pieces of soft plastic tubing or pipe insulation at a hardware store in various sizes and slip them over the old handles. Ask the clerk at the store to cut them into the lengths you need.

Sit higher. Maneuvering into and out of a chair can be a challenge. One quick way to make it easier is to raise the seat. Insert a firm pillow under the bottom cushion or in the seat of the chair. You'll find you're that much closer to "landing" when you go to sit down and have less far to go when you get up again.

Adapt your wardrobe. Avoid buying clothes with back zippers or multiple buttons. And for favorite garments, consider asking a tailor to replace buttons with hook-and-loop material (such as Velcro) or snaps.

Grab bars. Hoisting yourself out of a tub or even a shower can be difficult. A well-placed grab bar to help pull yourself up or just steady yourself can be a tremendous boon. Or, if you plan to renovate your bathroom, you may want to choose a walk-in shower or one with a built-in seat so that you can shower while sitting. Don't forget the vital nonslip mat, too, if you don't already have one.

USING SPLINTS AND OTHER SUPPORTS

A splint is a device made of cloth, plastic, or metal that straps onto a joint to keep it immobile. Splints are made for wrists, neck, fingers, hands, back, knees, and ankles. They help you by preventing your joint from moving while it is inflamed, which both eases pain and helps keep you from damaging the joint. A splint should be light enough that you can wear it comfortably and continue to do range-of-motion exercises.

Ready-made splints may fill the bill, or you may need custom-made ones. These are made "on the spot" by a physical or occupational therapist from plastics that are molded to fit your joint and then attached with Velcro straps.

While a splint can be useful to rest or protect your joints, using one too often can weaken and stiffen joints and thus limit their flexibility. Your best bet, doctors say, is to use a splint only during flare-ups and remove it several times a day to put your joint through some range-of-motion exercises.

If you need to use a cane, crutches, or walker, be sure that your doctor or physical therapist shows you how to use it properly to avoid further harm to the joint. A cane, for example, should be held in the hand opposite the painful joint. It should fit right, too: When you're standing up, the top of the cane should come to the crease inside your elbow, between the wrist and the upper arm.

Sometimes keeping your independence means easing up on your "image." Canes, crutches, and walkers can help you get around. Some people are hesitant or stubborn about using these supportive devices in the mistaken belief it makes them look "old." Try a new thought on for size: They make you look determined and gutsy. If a cane can help save a joint or relieve pain, don't hesitate to use one. You can find a comfortable plain variety at the drugstore or have a little fun with it by shopping around for a more decorative model for flair. And it may cheer you to know that if your doctor writes a prescription or recommendation for these devices, your insurance company may pay all or part of the cost.

WHEN AND HOW TO USE SPLINTS

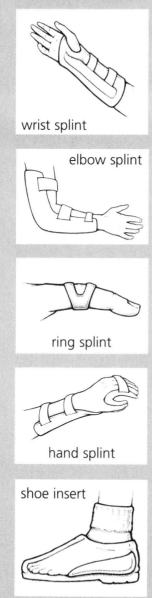

wrist splint

elbow splint

ring splint

hand splint

shoe insert

Splints are strap-on supports used to immobilize joints during bouts of inflammation. Fashioned from plastic, cloth, or metal, these devices provide joint stability, pain relief, and protection from injury. You're most likely to benefit from custom-made splints designed by a physical or occupational therapist or a prosthetics specialist. A material called orthroplast is heated until it is flexible, and then molded around the affected joint into a well-fitting and comfortable shape. The splint is then immersed in cold water until it sets. Some models can be slipped on, while others are fitted with Velcro or other easy-to-manage straps. Several different varieties are shown here.

Splints can be remarkably effective for resting and protecting inflamed joints, especially the wrists and fingers, and may also improve function in a severely damaged joint. However, incorrect or extended use can worsen joint stiffness, decrease strength, and limit flexibility. Thus, splints should only be used during painful flare-ups, and even then, should be removed several times a day to perform some gentle range-of-motion exercises.

YOU'RE NOT ALONE

It can be a little too easy to slip into depression when you're fighting a disease such as arthritis. You may not be able to garden all day, go hiking with your friends, or even fix the fancy dinners you used to love preparing for special occasions. You may have unpleasant reactions to the medications you are taking. In fact, you may both look and feel so different that you hardly feel like yourself.

If you begin to feel blue or just begin to have trouble coping with your health problems, realize that you aren't alone. There are caring people who can help and who have gone through this themselves. And there are professionals well versed in the problems you've encountered, who can offer invaluable advice and support. You may not be accustomed to sharing your troubles, but this isn't the time to be too proud to seek help or companionship.

Here are some ways to reach out:

- Talk to your doctor. Besides a sympathetic ear, your doctor may offer you a referral to an appropriate professional, prescribe antidepressant medication (as we discussed in chapter 3), or have good suggestions for supportive reading.

- Look in your newspaper's calendar section for arthritis support groups. Or you can find compassionate listeners even in support groups with another theme, such as Overeaters Anonymous or groups for retirees.

- Find a therapist. (See "Dealing with Depression," in chapter 3, for advice in locating a good therapist.) If you've never tried counseling, you'll be amazed at the comfort it can bring.

- Form your own group of friends with arthritis, who get together once a week for coffee at a member's home. You can share tips and coping strategies or just commiserate over cake. And don't forget the amazing ability of laughter to lift your spirits. Rent a comedy video, and celebrate some humor together.

- Check with your local YMCA or community center for classes, meetings, and trips for those with arthritis.
- Contact the Arthritis Foundation, a nonprofit organization that sponsors classes and produces books and a monthly magazine. (To contact the foundation, call 800-283-7800 or look up *http://www.arthritis.org* on the Internet.) You can request pamphlets or other information both from your computer and over the phone.

FINDING THE RIGHT SHOES AND ORTHOTICS

If you have rheumatoid arthritis in your feet, it's crucial to find shoes that fit well and protect your feet and ankles. They should be light and made of a breathable material such as leather or canvas, with good shock absorption and a stiff back. If you wear shoes with heels, they should be no higher than one inch.

Orthotics is a fancy name for special inserts that make shoes fit better and support your feet. The best kind are custom-made for you by a podiatrist, orthotist, or pedorthist. Orthotics help because they spread your weight more evenly over your foot rather than allowing it to be concentrated in one place.

If the shape of your feet has changed from arthritis, you may need specially made shoes. Your doctor can steer you to a specialty shoemaker. Custom-made shoes are more expensive than regular shoes, of course, so check to see if your insurance will cover part of the cost.

To help avoid problems, keep your feet clean, with nails trimmed straight across. Watch for blisters and calluses, and treat them right away if they appear. Pad blisters with moleskin pads available from the drugstore, and apply antibiotic ointment if the skin tears. For calluses, treat your feet to a 15-minute soak, then file down the callus gently with an emery board. (Never attempt to treat foot problems yourself if you are diabetic, however.)

ARTHRITIS AND YOUR LOVE LIFE

When your joints are aching or certain positions are painful, you may find yourself seldom if ever in the mood for sex. You could decide to give up on the whole idea, but this is rarely the best answer. A warm and loving sexual side to your relationship can add comfort and great pleasure to your life—and your partner's—and giving it up can be hard on both of you.

The first step is to talk to your partner and explain the problems you are having. Now is no time for reticence. You may be able to change positions slightly or spend more time in foreplay. Something as simple as placing a pillow under your hips can erase some of the strain, or you may find that making love while on your side is the most comfortable position. The Arthritis Foundation publishes a free "Living and Loving" guide, which offers detailed help, including specific alternate positions for particular kinds of aches and pains. (Call 800-283-7800, or order the guide over the Internet at *http://www.arthritis.org*.)

Plan romance for those times of the day when you have the least pain and the most energy. You also may find it more comfortable to take a warm bath first or to warm up the sheets with an electric blanket.

RETHINK YOUR ROUTINES

When rheumatoid arthritis or another inflammatory disease flares up, every little move can hurt—and can even damage your joints. You need to be smart about using your body. You can make every motion count and reduce pain by approaching your tasks more efficiently.

Think about how to minimize strain on your body: Every little bit helps, sometimes more than you may think possible. Remember, the world won't end if you relax your standards. The choice is clear: Immaculate house, buzz-cut lawn and aching joints? Or a less perfect environment and less pain? Here are some tips to aid day-to-day living.

In the Kitchen and Laundry Room

Lighten your daily routine. This is another time to examine what "image" might be costing you. Ask yourself if daily vacuuming is really important to your happiness. Or, if you're a die-hard housekeeper, now's the time to splurge and get yourself that new lightweight vacuum you've been admiring in the ads. Yes, it really does make a difference pushing this light machine rather than your old clunky one. Likewise, replace your iron with a lighter model, or better yet, put shirts on hangers to dry and give up ironing completely! If you have heavy or earthenware dishes, consider getting a cheerful but lightweight set for everyday use.

Spare your fingers. Tie or loop strips of cloth around drawer handles and the refrigerator door, so you can pull them open with your arm and not your hand. Use your palm to open jars, or invest in a specialized can opener for people with arthritis. Seal plastic containers with your elbow, not your thumb or fingers. (You can order special can openers and such from the Arthritis Foundation at 800-283-7800.)

Don't stretch. Before your arthritis hit, you may have routinely strained to get things out of a top cupboard or reached over the washing machine to the overhead cupboards without a thought about it. You can relearn these habits. Rearrange your cupboards so that the items you need most often are stored within easy reach. When you must get items from high shelves, use a sturdy step stool.

For cooking on that back burner, use long-handled utensils to stir instead of reaching over. Use long-handled wooden tongs to pick up items you can't reach easily and to retrieve clothes from the dryer.

Protect your back. When you're shopping, tote your bags in a small, foldable cart. If you must lift something, bend your knees and not your back. (But remember, when your knees are bothering you, it's best not to lift at all.)

Slide, don't lift. Whenever possible, slide objects instead of picking them up.

Throughout the House

Take a good look at your furniture. If you're like many of us, your house has practically filled up on its own over the years, without much rhyme or reason. You've added pieces of furniture where they fit, maybe squeezing in a couch your neighbor was giving away or stashing a beloved old armchair in the corner of the living room. Or perhaps you're the opposite: You have a keen sense of decor and your home is lovingly, elegantly furnished. Either way, now it's time to look at your home with new eyes. Is it difficult to get around because of too much furniture? Take a deep breath and either call Goodwill or have some items moved to storage. When you get out of bed at night, do you have to circumvent several things on your way to the bathroom? Clear your path. If your mattress is ancient and mushy, take yourself off to the mattress store: You need a firm mattress, and you may want an egg crate foam pad on top for extra comfort. Move chairs with arms into your favorite spots. These are much easier to get into and out of.

Change your doorknobs. This relatively inexpensive change can make day-to-day life much easier. Instead of round doorknobs that can be difficult to grip, choose the lever variety that need only to be lightly pushed.

Slip-proof your house. Scatter rugs may be attractive, but they're easy to slip on and sometimes hard to vacuum. And, if you're using a cane or walker, they're catastrophes waiting to happen. Box them up or give them away.

Switch on, switch off. Swap your standard wall switches with the small toggle for new ones you can turn on and off by simply pushing or bumping them. Likewise, you may want to replace the lamps you use most often with those that you turn on and off with a touch anywhere on the base.

In the Bathroom

Change handles. The handles on regular water taps can be difficult to turn; have them replaced with lever handles you can lightly push on and off.

Tie up your soap. Leaning over to fish your slippery soap off the tub or shower floor is not a good idea. You can mount a dispenser on the wall, filled with liquid soap you dispense with a push, or try soap on a rope, decorative soap with a long cord loop through the center. These can be hung over your arm or around your neck for easy retrieval.

Try a whirlpool. When it comes time for remodeling, you may want to consider installing a whirlpool bath, which can give lovely relief to aching limbs. Of course, you'll want to include a handrail on the side of the tub.

Walk into your shower. If it's possible, install a walk-in shower, one with a seat so you can shower while resting your legs. Or use a sturdy portable bath stool.

DAY-TO-DAY LIVING MADE EASIER

And there's still more you can do:

Go for automatic. If your car doesn't have an automatic transmission, now's the time to make the switch. Likewise, here's the case for that automatic garage door opener you've always wanted.

Get a permit. When you have arthritis, walking from the far end of the mall parking lot is not a good idea. While you may dislike the term, you're one of the people those reserved "handicapped" parking spaces are set aside for. Apply at your motor vehicle bureau for a handicapped parking license or sticker. You will likely need a form or note from your doctor, so call the bureau first to ask for details.

Change your job description. Especially if you've been together for a while, you and your mate probably have a clear split of duties. One cooks; one does dishes. One mops; one dusts. One changes the oil; one washes the car. These vary for everyone, but the point is that you may need to change your pattern when one partner has arthritis and the other doesn't. You may not be fond of changing the status quo—or even admitting that certain tasks pain you—but marriage is a partnership, which means sharing what comes to us in life. Talk to your spouse and explain the problem. You may even find that you both enjoy doing different "jobs" for a change.

Get help. Now may be the time—especially during painful flare-ups. Empty out your spare-change stash and hire a neighbor teen to mow the lawn. Call a maid service to do your spring cleaning. Take your car to be washed instead of doing it by hand. Spend what you can to spare your joints, and save your energy for things that are more fun.

Think ahead. Before you do even small tasks, think them through. You want to avoid jarring, bouncing, painful movements and during flare-ups, minimize all movement. If you're cooking, put all the ingredients in one spot (and, of course, you've already arranged those cupboards so that items you use often are together in the first place). Ask yourself, "What's the least stressful way I can do this?"

Change positions often. One of the worst things you can do for yourself is to sit or stand in one position. Keep shifting about so that you don't stiffen up.

Use the largest joint possible. If you're holding a cup of tea, use your palms, not your fingers. If you're pushing a door open, use your shoulder or buttocks, not your wrist.

Keep warm. Getting chilled seems to make arthritic joints ache, so keep yourself toasty. Dress in layers to keep your joints warm. Have leaky windows sealed up. If your favorite chair is under an air vent, have it moved.

Protect your hands. Wear your purse or tote bag across your shoulder instead of lugging it in your hands. If you must carry heavy objects, hold them with both arms close to your body.

Plan ascents and descents. If you have one leg that's stronger or less painful, start up the stairs with that leg, and start down with the same one. Always use a handrail (and be sure you have rails on all the steps in and near your home, including the porches). If you have serious problems with stairs, consider installing stair lifts in your home or moving your bedroom to the first floor. Some people who move from a two- or three-story house to a one-level house find that life's a lot easier.

MAKE SOME CHANGES AT WORK

Many of us have workplaces that were, well, thrown together rather than designed. A regular desk has been converted to hold a desktop computer. Filing cabinets have been added as needed. Older files may be kept in bins on top of the file cabinets. Tools may be scattered about.

For joint health—and especially if you have rheumatoid arthritis—you can't afford such a haphazard layout for a place in which you spend 40 or more hours a week.

THREE GREAT TIPS FOR EVERY DAY

There are three small things you can do that will make your day-to-day life infinitely easier.

Roll out of bed. You've probably been getting out of bed the same way just about every day of your life. Chances are you fling back the covers, swing your legs out, sit up, and then stand. Essentially, you're doing a sit-up from your bed. If you have any arthritis pain in your back, what works better is to first roll to your side and then use your arms to carefully hoist yourself up.

Get the right kind of chair. If you have any pain in your back, replace your armless chairs with ones with arms. The additional support will help tremendously when you're getting up and down.

Lift the right way. When we drop a book on the floor, most of us bend over any which way. It's important, however, to lift even small things correctly. Bend at the knee, and grasp the object, if it's heavy at all, close to your body. Then lift with your legs, not your arms.

Protect your wrists. A painful wrist condition called carpal tunnel syndrome can result from repetitive motions such as typing on a keyboard. This pain is caused by pressure on the nerve where it passes through the carpal tunnel in the wrist. Buy a wrist support that sits in front of the keyboard. They're available at computer or office supply stores.

Use good mechanics. Just as you do at home, if you must stoop to lift objects, do so with your knees bent. Instead of pushing a door open with your hand, use your hip, shoulders, or upper arm.

Strive for comfort. Insist on a comfortable chair at work, with arms if possible and wheels to help you get around your place of business more easily. Adjust your chair height so your desk or work space is two inches below your elbow. If you work on cars or other machinery, use a stool with wheels, and choose lighter-weight tools whenever possible.

WHAT IF YOU GET PREGNANT?

If you have rheumatoid arthritis or another inflammatory disease such as lupus, you'll want to carefully think through the decision to have a child and plan thoroughly before the birth. Besides the strain of pregnancy, you'll also need to consider the physical demands of taking care of an infant and then a young child.

Medication for lupus presents a serious barrier. Although internal inflammation is rarely an issue in rheumatoid arthritis, if you do have inflammation in an internal organ or are required to take more than 10 milligrams of prednisone daily, your doctor will likely ask you to delay pregnancy until these problems abate. Unfortunately, although most women with rheumatoid arthritis actually feel better during pregnancy, the bottom line is that because of the risk of birth defects, if you are on medication it is best to avoid pregnancy unless your doctor has given you the go-ahead.

If you do conceive, you will likely work with a rheumatologist and an obstetrician-gynecologist and possibly a maternal fetal specialist. Although pregnancy has its discomforts for every woman, you may need to also prepare for other changes:

- Your joints may loosen.
- Knee problems may become worse.
- You may get muscle spasms in your back and sometimes pain or numbness and tingling in your legs.
- You may retain water, which can increase stiffness and make carpal tunnel syndrome worse.

Ask about your medications. Your doctor may shift you to less toxic medicines during your pregnancy or decrease the doses. Generally, aspirin and prednisone can be used cautiously during pregnancy. The drugs penicillamine, methotrexate, cyclophosphamide (Cytoxan), and azathioprine (Imuran) must be avoided because of the chance of birth defects. Do not, however, change any medications on your own. You should also discuss with your doctor any other medications you are taking, including over-the-counter preparations.

Consider your milk. Medicines you take may be passed to the baby via breast milk. It will help to take your medicines after your baby has eaten in the morning, so she won't be taking in as much. Talk to your doctors. You may choose to alternate breast feeding with formula to limit the amount of medication your baby receives.

Reconsider exercise. Exercise is recommended for pregnant women, but if you have an inflammatory disease, you may be considered high risk, especially if you have an accompanying condition such as heart complications, inflammation of the veins, or high blood pressure. So it's crucial to discuss your exercise program with your doctor. He may ask you to switch to a different type of exercise or give you guidelines on limiting your activity. (It's a good idea to get into shape *before* getting pregnant so that you have strong quadriceps muscles, the large ones above your knees. These provide better support for your joints.)

Watch your weight gain. Generally, women should gain between 20 and 30 pounds during pregnancy. Too much, and you'll overtax your joints. Too little, and the baby may not get enough nutrients. Ask your doctor what the best overall weight gain is for you specifically and how much you should gain each month.

CHANGING YOUR OUTLOOK

Arthritis, by its very nature, induces stress: It changes the familiar patterns of your life; it can make you feel as though you have little control. You hurt, you can't do all the things you used to do, and you may even look somewhat different.

Sometimes people give up activities simply because they can no longer do them at their accustomed pace. A better solution is to approach the activity in a new way: If going out for dinner exhausts you, go out for coffee instead. If you desperately miss dancing, try a single dance or slow dancing, or sign up for a class in t'ai chi, a graceful and dancelike (but non-impact) Chinese art. Return to your weight-lifting program by starting off with very light weights and gradually increasing them as your joints permit.

In some cases, you may have to shift your sights to reinvolve yourself in a beloved pastime. This also works with less appealing activities such as housework.

Researchers have found that most of us can cope pretty well with things as long as we believe we have the resources to handle them. It's when we conclude that the problems are beyond our capacity to manage that stress takes over. So the ticket here, as clichéd as it sounds, is to think positively. Not only can this make you feel better emotionally, but it will make you feel better physically, too.

Dealing with pain itself can be emotionally debilitating. Without realizing it, you can make the pain worse by tensing up, anticipating and dreading it. If you think, "This is going to hurt," before you get up, you're basically priming the pump for pain. And fear can actually increase its severity.

Likewise, feelings of worthlessness, a sense of guilt at slowing down your partner, or negative thoughts such as, "No one understands what I'm going through," increase the likelihood that you're going to feel rotten both mentally and physically.

Pain may seem straightforward, but it's not that simple. There's a "gate control" theory of pain that helps explain why soldiers wounded in battle may feel little or no pain when it happens, while amputees may feel excruciating agony in limbs that are no longer even there. The idea is that you have a nerve "gate" in your spine. When something hurts, the nervous system sends pain signals toward the brain through the spinal cord. If the gate is open, the pain signal gets through; if it's closed, it doesn't.

And believe it or not, what you *feel* and *think* has been proven to affect the opening or closing of this gate.

CHAPTER 10

An Exercise Program for You

One of the best things you can do for your joints is to use them—carefully, that is. Joints need consistent, gentle movement to help keep the cartilage healthy and the joint mobile. If you don't regularly move a joint, it can stiffen or even "freeze" when your muscles and tendons become too weak or tight.

Staying active is one of the best things you can do for your joints (and your heart and lungs, too). Regular exercise, whether swimming, weight training, walking, or another type of gentle workout, can help rejuvenate joints that have become a bit creaky.

And most people with arthritis don't exercise enough. A review from the Centers for Disease Control and Prevention found that more than a third of those with arthritis didn't exercise regularly, and that's less than the general population. Even when they did exercise, people with arthritis were less likely to do the recommended minimum of 20 minutes at a time, three days a week.

One of the best ways to protect your cartilage from damage is through *controlled* movement: moving easily and correctly. Otherwise, you can overstress your joints with poor mechanics—holding your neck at an awkward angle to look at a computer monitor, for example, or even just having poor posture. Good balance and coordination can help even out the stresses placed on your joints, however, and a workout program can help you develop and keep these traits.

If you have rheumatoid arthritis, of course, you should not exercise during a flare-up—except for a gentle range-of-motion routine, if you feel up to it. But when the inflammation subsides, you will want to ease into a workout program to begin building your strength. If you have significant damage from osteoarthritis, you'll need to select gentle activities that won't further damage your joint, such as swimming, water aerobics, or bicycling.

PLANNING YOUR ATTACK

All the activities we're about to discuss can help you create a more mobile and less painful life. Although all of these are relatively "gentle" exercises that don't place undue stress on your joints, you should still clear any exercise with your doctor and your physical therapist, if you have one. They may suggest steering clear of certain moves that might aggravate your condition or recommend a specific exercise that suits your needs best.

If you've been inactive or are starting a new kind of exercise, the most important thing is to start slowly and increase your activity levels slowly. Try to increase by no more than 10 percent a week. If you walk a mile comfortably every day this week, for example, try a mile plus a tenth next week.

How do you know what activity to choose? Think about the things you used to do "B.A."—before arthritis. Consider how much free time you have, if you want to exercise at home, in a gym, or on the open road, and how much money you want to spend. Consult your doctor first, of course, and choose an activity that puts the least stress on your damaged or painful joints.

You may also want to consider cross-training, which means alternating activities so you don't overtax one set of muscles or joints. If you're a fitness walker, substitute a swim once a week, for example, or if you take yoga classes, enjoy a bike ride.

Just keep moving whenever you can!

WORKING OUT
WITH YOUR PHYSICAL THERAPIST

Maybe you've tried to start working out on your own, but every time, you get sore and discouraged and drop out. This time, see your physical therapist before you begin. Physical therapists *specialize* in developing gradual and varied programs aimed at keeping you healthy—and keeping you at it.

To start, your physical therapist will interview you or ask you to fill out a questionnaire, including questions about any limitations you have, what types of activities you like, and what times of the day are convenient for exercise.

Next comes testing to determine your capabilities. This might include a treadmill or step test or muscle testing on exercise equipment. Your balance and coordination may also be checked, as well as your posture and how mobile your joints are.

Now the physical therapist sets up your individual exercise plan, which will include a variety of activities and exercises, tailored to your needs, likes, and dislikes. If you're interested in buying an exercise machine, your physical therapist can recommend equipment that will work well for you.

You'll be taught how to warm up and cool down and how to check your pulse and breathing rate. Your physical therapist likely will ask you to keep a simple log of your activities, which includes noting how you feel. On the basis of this log, your physical therapist may modify your program so that it suits you even better.

ALL ABOUT WALKING

You love to walk to the corner store, but it's becoming more and more painful. As gentle as walking may seem, it is a weight-bearing exercise. When you walk, you're putting your full body weight on your hips, knees, and ankles, step after step. And if you're overweight, you're putting more stress on those joints than they're designed for.

If you have significant osteoarthritis, your doctor may advise you to limit your walking. But if your osteoarthritis is minor or you have another type of arthritis that will permit walking, it can be a great and enjoyable exercise.

The right gear. The most crucial thing you can do to help yourself build a successful walking program is to buy good shoes. The shoes you have may look fine on top, but often the soles have worn unevenly or the cushioning material inside the shoe, where you can't see has collapsed. Yes, athletic shoes can be expensive, but think of them as an investment in your joints. Go to a sports shoe store and explain to the clerk that you need good walking shoes. Consider trying the kind with air or gel in the soles that give you extra cushioning, and replace them every 500 miles.

Getting started. Try walking 10 minutes at a time, five days a week, at first. Next week, add another 5 minutes. If that's comfortable, continue to add 5 minutes a week until you've gotten up to at least 25 minutes.

Stand erect, with your shoulders back and your head held high. Let your arms swing freely. Generally, you'll want to walk in a gentle heel-toe motion, although doctors may advise some people with arthritis to put their whole foot down—gently. Never slam your foot against the ground.

Perhaps you like to walk around the neighborhood circle, four laps a night, or you may prefer the high school track's nice smooth surface. Great idea, but most roads or tracks are cambered, or slanted, in one direction, so you'll be putting slightly more stress on one leg with each step. That doesn't sound dire, but it can add up. The solution is easy: Just walk in the other direction every other session!

Summary: Moderate stress on ankles, knees, hips, and spine.

ALL ABOUT STRETCHING

Often a gentle daily stretching routine can make the difference between having joints that work smoothly and ones that don't. You may not notice that you've cut back on your level of activity. Then one day you realize that you can no longer reach up to the top shelf of your hall closet or that stooping to look through a bottom drawer is painful.

Although it may seem that these difficulties crept up overnight, it can take years of neglect or misuse before you feel much pain or notice that a joint is not cooperating. Often people will say, "I don't know what happened; suddenly I just had this pain." But physical therapists often say that after watching how people move and listening to them describe what they do during the day, it's clear that problems had been building up for years.

So keep those joints stretched out! Inflexibility makes you more prone to injury. And because everything in your body is connected, pain doesn't always show up in the troublesome joint. A stiff knee may be influenced by ankle or hip problems, for instance. Or an inflexible neck can trigger shoulder pain. A tennis player may feel pain on the outside of the arm, often called tennis elbow, but the actual problem may be an inflexible shoulder that causes the player to extend the elbow too far or "snap" the wrist.

How can you regain mobility in the joints you've neglected or head off joint problems if none have yet started? Build stretching and activity into your daily lifestyle.

Run every joint through its natural range of motion as often as possible. If you have a dog or cat, look at how often it stretches, and imitate Fido or Tiger.

You may find a low-impact exercise video useful, but first you should clear the tape with your doctor or physical therapist. Some routines are too stressful for people with joint problems.

Stretch whenever it's most comfortable for you. Often it's best to stretch after light activity has warmed up your muscles. You may find it easier while in the shower or bath or in bed, where it's nice and warm. Generally, hold stretches for 15 to 20 seconds; stretch gently and never bounce or force it. Stretching also should be part of your warm-up and cool down routine for other physical activities.

The following sections describe stretching exercises for specific parts of the body.

Neck and Shoulders

- Throughout the day, move your head from side to side as if trying to look behind you. Then, look up at the ceiling and down at your feet.
- Stretch out your shoulders. Stand next to a doorway with your arm against the door in the shape of an **L**. Slowly twist your upper body until you feel a gentle pull in your shoulder muscles. Repeat with the other arm.
- Reach your arms up to the ceiling, one at a time. Then reach down and pat yourself on the back. Another good stretch is to slowly shrug your shoulders. You can do these at your desk or while watching television.
- Check your posture: Stand naturally and comfortably in front of a full-length mirror and take a look. If your shoulders and head are slumping forward, imagine a string on the top of your head tugging you erect.

Wrists and Fingers

- Take one hand at a time and bend the wrist slowly forward and back, then make a loose fist and slowly stretch your fingers out straight. Repeat with the other hand. To keep your fingers strong, squeeze a tennis ball or racquetball.
- Put your hands in a "praying" position, and try to bend your wrists so that your arms form a straight line to the elbows. Or hold your hand flat on your desk and slowly bring your arm forward over it until you feel the stretch in your wrist and forearm.

Arms

- Stick out your arm with the palm down, and then use your other hand to gently pull up on the wrist. Hold 10 seconds, repeat five times, and then repeat for the other arm.

Knees

- Lie on the floor beside a doorway. Place one leg up against the wall with the heel on the wall and the knee straight, and leave the other leg lying on the floor through the doorway. Inch yourself closer to the wall until you feel the stretch. Repeat with the other leg.
- Stand facing a wall, bracing yourself with your hands. With a small ankle weight, slowly lift your foot behind you until your shin is parallel with the floor. Hold for 10 seconds, then lower the foot. Repeat 10 times for each foot.

Calves

- Stand near a wall with one foot about 12 inches from the wall and the other foot another 12 inches behind that. With both feet flat on the floor, place your arms about shoulder height and lean forward, keeping the back leg straight and bending the front knee. Repeat with your other leg. Then repeat with both knees bent.

- To stretch out the front of your knee, lie on your front. Bend one knee and gently pull your heel toward your buttocks. Repeat with your other leg.
- To stretch your iliotibial band, an important muscle that runs down the outside of the thigh and connects to the leg bone below the kneecap, stand with your right side toward the wall and put your right hand against the wall at shoulder level. Cross your left leg over the right leg and lean your hip gently toward the wall. Repeat for the other side.

Hips

- Lie flat on your back and gently pull your left thigh toward your chest, while keeping your back flat. Repeat for the other leg.
- Stand with your legs wide apart and twist your upper body gently so that you feel a pull on your upper inner leg.
- Sit on the ground with your knees bent and the bottoms of your feet together and as close to your body as is comfortable. Put your hands on your knees and push down gently.
- Sit on the ground with one leg flat and the other bent at the knee. Cross the bent leg over the straight leg and gently pull the knee toward your chest. Repeat with the other leg.

Ankles

- Sit with your foot hanging, then rotate your ankle in circles 10 times. Repeat in the other direction; then repeat for the other foot.

ALL ABOUT SWIMMING

Swimming gives your muscles, heart, and lungs a great workout. When one group of previously inactive middle-aged adults swam for 12 weeks, their oxygen uptake increased an average of 20 percent, and their hearts pumped more blood with each beat.

The great thing about swimming is that the buoyancy of the water essentially carries your body weight. And your heart rate is lower in swimming than in other sports. It's the ideal exercise for people with arthritis and joint problems (and it's good for anyone who goes with you, too).

The right gear. To liven up your pool workouts, you may want to use fins. These make your legs work in both directions, using your thigh, calf, and abdominal muscles, and keep you from overworking your arms and shoulders. They're also helpful when recovering from knee injuries.

You could also use a pull-buoy, which is two Styrofoam cylinders held together with cords. You place it between your thighs, and it holds your lower body up in the water, letting you paddle without kicking. And try a kickboard, a flat piece of Styrofoam you hang on to so that you can kick without paddling or arm strokes. Hand paddles and webbed gloves are designed to help strengthen your arms, but because they increase the risk of shoulder problems, steer clear.

If you're troubled by swimmer's ear (a bacterial or fungal infection caused when water washes away protective earwax), you may want to use earplugs. You can also swab your ears with alcohol after swimming or use an over-the-counter preparation of alcohol or glycerin drops.

Getting started. If you find yourself gasping for breath after one lap, you probably aren't going to be eager to swim again. The trick is to get in shape first. Walk or use a stationary bicycle so that you'll be fit enough to stay in the water longer when you do climb in. And stretch before swimming, in the pool or out. This warms up your muscles to increase blood flow and flexibility. You could walk or jog in place in the water or stretch while holding on to the side of the pool. Next comes light swimming to warm up for a few minutes.

If all you can do at first is stretch, warm up, paddle a lap, and then cool down, then that's what you should do. Don't force yourself through a painful or exhausting workout: If you're tired, you're going to get hurt.

Likewise, if swimming is tiring, you may need to improve your style. Swimming incorrectly can tire you or strain your muscles. You also may want to learn different strokes to make your pool time more interesting. You can sign up for lessons or join a masters' swim group for coaching.

Realize that swimming in too-cold water causes you to lose too much heat and stresses your cardiovascular system. Too-warm water overheats you and also stresses your system.

Many pools are kept at 70 to 73 degrees, which requires you to move briskly to stay warm. (Wearing two swimsuits, one atop the other, and a swim cap can help.) Most of us can swim comfortably in temperatures of 82 to 86 degrees, but the 92- to 98-degree temperature of therapeutic pools is designed for limited movement only and is too warm for swimming.

Summary: Mild stress on elbows, shoulders, and spine.

ALL ABOUT WATER WORKOUTS

Remember doing calisthenics in high school? Or maybe you have grim memories of aerobics classes where you were doggedly leaping about, always one step behind and definitely not having fun.

Exercising in water is a whole new experience and most people with arthritis love it. You don't need any special skills, and with certain simple equipment, you don't even need to know how to swim. All you need is water. The natural buoyancy of the water aids movement, letting you do exercises that might be too painful or stressful on land.

Water exercise covers a wide range of activities: water aerobics, supervised sessions prescribed by a physical therapist, or running or doing jumping jacks in your backyard pool. It can be done with your head completely above water or can include bobbing or rolling in water. It can be done in deep or shallow water, in a regular pool, or in a heated therapeutic facility.

And water is a great place to work out. Water effectively reduces your body weight by 90 percent. So if you weigh 150 pounds, in water your limbs only have to support 15 pounds. Stress on joints, bones, and muscles is kept to a minimum.

Water can also help cool you off as you exercise, and any stiffness or pain you may be feeling may decrease. In heated or therapeutic pools there's no cooling effect, but the warm water helps relieve the pain of stiff joints or injured limbs.

And because water provides resistance to movement, pushing to move through it can tone and strengthen muscles and improve your range of motion. You get benefits similar to those from doing the exercises on land but with none of the jarring or pounding.

The right gear. If you can't swim, you may want to use a flotation vest, which also comes in handy for certain exercises. If you walk or jog in the pool, for example, the vest will keep you upright so that you don't have to struggle to keep your balance. Or you can use it in deeper water to keep an injured foot or ankle completely off the pool floor. You may also want fins, a pull-buoy, or a kickboard to vary your routine.

Getting started. Once your doctor has given the okay, you can sign up for a class at the community pool or devise your own workout. If you have a physical therapist, your therapist will design a program for you.

Whatever your program, spend five minutes warming up to get your body ready. You can warm up in the pool or in a whirlpool or hot tub. You can sit on the edge of the pool and do flutter kicks and circle your feet in the water. Or, while you're in the pool, jog in place or do other stretches.

A good beginning water exercise session might include a 5-minute warm-up, 10-minute workout, and 5-minute cooldown, three times a week. Another workout you can do on your own is pool walking or jogging. After a warm-up, spend 10 to 20 minutes traveling back and forth from one end of the pool to the other. For variety, try walking sideways or backwards. If the pool bottom is slippery, wear a pair of rubber-soled water socks or water sandals.

Remember, for most pool exercises, a good temperature range is 82 to 86 degrees.

Summary: Mild stress on ankles, knees, hips, elbows, shoulders, spine.

ALL ABOUT BICYCLING

Bicycling doesn't pound your lower joints as jogging or even brisk walking can, because much of your weight is supported by the bicycle seat. This makes biking particularly good for people who are overweight or have some joint damage. People with osteoarthritis in bicycling programs not only improved muscle strength and aerobic capacity, but also reduced their joint pain and fatigue.

The right gear. An old bike may do just fine (after a quick tune-up). Be sure to adjust the saddle height, because riding with it too high or too low can cause joint problems. There should be only a slight bend in your knee when pedaling with the balls of your feet. If you're rocking from side to side as you pedal, the saddle is too high; if your knee is bent quite a bit, it's too low.

You can buy gel-pad-filled saddle covers if the saddle is too hard, and you may be more comfortable on wider saddles (women's "sit" bones are farther apart than men's). You can ride in any comfortable clothes, but you may want to consider the additional comfort of bike shorts with a padded, seamless crotch. (If you ride in long pants, wrap a rubber band loosely around the right pants leg so that it doesn't get caught up in the chain, or buy bike clips made for that purpose.) Padded, fingerless bike gloves will keep your hands from getting numb and protect your palms in case you take a tumble. And a helmet is a must. Some folks can ride in regular sneakers with no problems, but if you find your feet getting numb, head to the bike store and check out bike shoes with stiff soles that spread the pressure around.

Getting started. When you're just starting, you may want to limit yourself to jaunts around your neighborhood. Specifically, stay away from hills. A beginner may want to ride 10 minutes at a time, three times a week, and increase that by 5 minutes each week.

Don't make the mistake of pushing a high gear, which forces you to pedal slowly. This is inefficient and can cause knee and muscle pain. You're much better off in a lower gear, spinning the pedals faster. Pedal with the balls of your feet, never your heels or insteps.

Glance at your watch or have someone time you for 60 seconds and count the number of times you turn the pedals over in one minute. Sixty or more revolutions per minute is the most efficient pace and least likely to cause injury.

Your goal may be to ride 20 minutes three times a week. Warm up the first three to five minutes and end with a three- to five-minute cooldown by riding slowly in an easy gear. As your fitness level increases, you can increase the time you ride.

If you're troubled by inflexibility or find yourself tightening up from cycling, start stretching out after your workout, specifically your hamstrings, calves, and quadriceps. Don't stretch before riding, when your muscles are cold.

Riding indoors. If you'd rather cycle indoors, you have plenty of choices. You can put a regular bike on an apparatus called a wind trainer, or you can use one of many varieties of stationary bicycle. Many people find models with seat backs more comfortable, and others prefer recumbent or semi-recumbent ones that you pedal with your legs in front of you. These bikes are less likely to cause pain in the buttocks and lower back and are often easier to climb onto.

In general, you want the smoothest, quietest ride and sturdiest bike possible, and a small digital panel that lets you track your workouts, preferably one that shows distance covered, speed, time, and how many calories you're burning. You can start indoors with a similar schedule to regular biking, at first setting the control for very little resistance.

You can get a magazine rack to prop up your favorite reading material or a headset with music to exercise by. And lots of people enjoy watching television while they pedal.

Summary: Outdoor biking—mild stress on the ankles, wrists, elbows, shoulders and spine and moderate stress on the knees and hips; stationary biking—mild stress on the ankle and spine; moderate stress on the knees and hips.

ALL ABOUT WEIGHT LIFTING

What can weight lifting do for you? More than you'd imagine. And you don't have to be Miss Universe or Arnold Schwarzenegger, either.

It doesn't matter how old you are or what degree of conditioning you're in. Weight lifting can help increase bone density and slow the loss of bone, lessening the risk of osteoporosis (which is heightened in people with arthritis who take corticosteroids). It can strengthen your joints and the surrounding ligaments, tendons and muscles, make losing weight easier, and, in many cases, improve your general sense of well-being.

In one study at Harvard, 90-year-olds who hadn't been able to walk unaided for years regained amazing amounts of mobility after a 10-week supervised weight-lifting program. These elderly men and women lifted light weights three times a week.

The right gear. You need something to lift, of course. For some exercises, it can be just a can of food; for others, you can use resistance bands, large rubbery bands that are somewhat like inner tubes. For more serious weight lifting, you may want padded fingerless gloves or a weight belt. All are available at most sporting goods stores.

Getting started. You need your doctor's okay, of course. You may also find it easier to work with a physical therapist or a trainer who knows your physical limitations. And it's a good plan to work out with weights only every other day or three times a week to allow your muscles time to recover from the deliberate pressure weight-lifting uses to strengthen them. You should start easily, perhaps just doing four of these exercises the first day and gradually adding more each week. Build up slowly.

Here are a few sample exercises you can do at home:

- To strengthen your shoulder's rotator cuff, the muscles connected to the joint capsule: Stand straight with a small weight in one hand (such as a can of food) and lift it in front of you until your arm is parallel with the floor. Repeat 5 to 10 times, then with the other arm. Then repeat again, this time lifting your arms straight out from your sides.

- To strengthen your triceps, the muscles in the back of your upper arms, hold a small weight behind your head, in both hands. Hold your upper arms still, and just extend your lower arms to lift the weight over your head. Repeat 5 to 10 times.

- To strengthen your biceps, those "Popeye" upper arm muscles, hold a weight in your hand, with your elbows at your sides. Slowly bend your elbow and raise the weight toward your chin. Repeat 5 to 10 times, and then do the other arm.

- To strengthen wrists, while seated, hold a small weight with your hand dangling free over your knee and your elbow propped on your leg. Curl your wrist up 10 times with the palm up, and then repeat with the palm down. Repeat for the other arm.

- To strengthen your quadriceps—the muscles in the front of your legs that let you straighten your knee and bend your leg at the hip—strap a small weight to your ankle and lift your leg straight out while seated (or you can do it without a weight, especially at first). Repeat 5 to 10 times for each leg.

Summary: Stress varies depending on exercise.

CHAPTER 11

The Future of Arthritis Treatment

There's no doubt about it—this is an exciting time for science when it comes to new treatments for arthritis.

For most forms of arthritis, treatment today centers on controlling the pain and limiting the damage. In some utopian future, hopefully not so far away, doctors may look back at our methods of dealing with arthritis as insignificant stopgaps. Instead, they may be routinely growing new cartilage for those of us with osteoarthritis and using our own immune systems to put rheumatoid arthritis on ice. Their goal is to stop osteoarthritis in its tracks and head off rheumatoid arthritis before it does any damage.

Right now, the medication you receive for osteoarthritis, whether prescription or over-the-counter, is mostly aimed at relieving your pain. But scientists are searching for a way to halt the breakdown of cartilage that causes the damage in the first place, and the future of osteoarthritis treatment will likely center on regrowing damaged cartilage.

For immune-based diseases such as rheumatoid arthritis, the goal is to learn more about the immune system and how to manipulate it. You can think of what goes wrong with your immune cells as the biological equivalent of police brutality: Some cop immune cells that are supposed to be fighting bad-guy germs are instead attacking normal citizens of your body—like your joints. Just a few "bad-cop" cells start the reaction that leads to the inflammation of these diseases, but current treatment involves "punishing" or suppressing *all* the cop immune cells. Scientists are learning more and more about how our bodies' police cells communicate with each other and hope that they'll be able to zero in on the bad-guy cells and develop treatments targeted at them alone.

Here's a closer look at what arthritis treatments of the future may include.

REPAIRING AND REPLACING CARTILAGE

As mentioned earlier in this book, cartilage is a living tissue, with cells that make new tissue and scavenge the old. In osteoarthritis, more cartilage is being broken down than is being formed. Researchers are now testing medications designed to alter this process so that the cartilage doesn't break down at all.

One of the most promising concepts is "growing" new cartilage to help replace the old. The idea is to take healthy cartilage cells from a knee, grow the cells in a culture, and then insert them like a patch in the damaged knee—sort of a "test tube" knee. The FDA approved a method called Carticel in 1996 as a safe way to regrow cartilage for people who have damage to the end of the thigh bone, near the top of the kneecap. This procedure is being performed at some medical centers in the United States, but for now it is mainly restricted to repairing small tears caused by injury. The procedure is astronomically expensive, and more research is needed before doctors know whether it will work for people with significant arthritis.

OTHER AREAS UNDER STUDY

A genetic link. While osteoarthritis doesn't have as strong a genetic link as inflammatory diseases do, genetic study is still underway. That's because doctors have discovered that a mutation in a collagen gene causes the production of defective cartilage in a certain group of people. People with this gene get osteoarthritis in their early 20s and need joint replacements decades sooner than they normally might. By studying this gene, scientists hope to figure out more about cartilage breakdown. The idea is that once you identify the gene that contributes to the breakdown of cartilage, you can try to figure out the whole process and how to stop it or slow it down.

Electric and magnetic therapy. You may have read that low-power magnetic fields or low-frequency electrical signals may help joints with osteoarthritis. These signals may encourage bone and cartilage to repair themselves or may just block the feeling of pain. However, this effect is not yet well understood or documented. And because there's no approved means of treatment with magnetism or electricity, anyone claiming to be able to cure you this way is operating without regulation and has no scientific guidelines to follow.

New medications ahead. Here's yet another acronym to remember: DMOAD, which stands for disease-modifying osteoarthritis drug. This is a type of medication, which includes tetracycline, tiaprofenic acid, and heparinoids. The idea is that DMOADs may stop the release of enzymes that damage cartilage. The drugs are being tested in animal studies.

Another group of drugs, cyclo-oxygenase-2 inhibitors, stops the inflammation of osteoarthritis. NSAIDs do much the same thing, but they also block an enzyme called cyclo-oxygenase-1, which protects the stomach lining. So if these new drugs work, they won't irritate your stomach as NSAIDs do. One such drug being tested by the FDA is celecoxib, a combination of diclofenac and misoprostol, which is manufactured under the brand name Arthtec.

UNLOCKING THE INFLAMMATION PUZZLE

Most treatments for rheumatoid arthritis involve controlling the immune system, because it's an immune response that causes the destructive inflammation. Of course, you need your immune system to fight off diseases and heal from injury. Unfortunately, however, most current treatments for inflammatory diseases block the beneficial immune responses as well. Ideally, arthritis medicines would block only the unwanted inflammation.

For a simpler way to understand the goals of current research, we'll look a little deeper into the police analogy, with a little help from Clint Eastwood. In one of the *Dirty Harry* movies, Eastwood's character comes to realize that a few cops have taken the law into their own hands and become the bad guys. In his typical "make my day" style, Harry quickly brings them to justice *without hurting any of the good cops.*

In the future, medical scientists will be able to do the same in fighting rheumatoid arthritis. They will be able to stop the "bad-cop" cells of our immune systems that are attacking the joints to cause rheumatoid arthritis. And, they will be able to leave the "good-cop" immune cells on the job, to continue protecting us from infection. This would be a great advantage because, as we've seen, current treatments tend to punish the entire immune system force— good- and bad-cop cells alike.

Doctors will be able to target treatments more effectively, because they will know much more about how to distinguish the many different cells in our immune systems. Just like a police department with its ranks of officers, the immune system contains more than one kind of cell. Not just good or bad cops, but some that work like cops patrolling the beat, and others that function more like sergeants.

So how do all these cells talk to each other? Researchers are also learning more about how the various cop cells communicate. The different immune cells use chemical substances called cytokines, which act more or less like radio signals. The more scientists learn how the cytokines function, the more possible it will become to devise treatments that "jam" signals to the bad-cop cells and put them out of business.

HOW TO KEEP UP WITH THE LATEST NEWS

Things are happening all the time in arthritis research. To keep abreast of late-breaking developments, to find more information or locate classes or books, contact the following:

Arthritis Foundation, 1314 Spring St. NW, Atlanta, GA 30309; 800-283-7800, 404-872-7100. The Internet address is *http://www.arthritis.org*.
The Foundation answers questions about arthritis, provides information about referrals, and offers:
- Self-help courses
- Water- and land-based exercise classes
- Support groups
- Home study courses
- Instructional videotapes
- Public forums
- Educational brochures and booklets
- A bimonthly magazine called *Arthritis Today*

You can order brochures and access fact sheets and more information on the Internet Web site at *http://www.arthritis.org* or contact your local chapter for class schedules.

American Academy of Orthopedic Surgeons, 6300 N. River Rd., Rosemont, IL 60018-4262; 800-346-AAOS; 708-823-7186. The Internet address is *http://www.aaos.org*.

American Lupus Society, 260 Maple Ct., Suite 124, Ventura, CA 93003; 800-331-1802; 805-339-0443.

Ankylosing Spondylitis Association, 511 N. La Cienga, #210, Los Angeles, CA 90048; 900-777-8189.

Arthritis Society, 250 Bloor St. E, Suite 901, Toronto, ONT, Canada M4W 3P2; 416-967-5679.

Johns Hopkins Vasculitis Center, 1830 E. Monument St., Room 7500, Baltimore, MD 21205. The Internet address is *http://vasculitis.med.jhu.edu*.

National Arthritis & Musculoskeletal & Skin Diseases Information Clearinghouse, One AMS Cir., Bethesda, MD 20892-3675; 301-495-4484.

National Fibromyalgia Research Association, Inc., Box 500, Salem, OR 97308.

National Institute on Aging Information Center, P.O. Box 8057, Gaithersburg, MD 20898-8057; 800-222-2225.